SUPERFOOD SHAKES

HOW TO GO BEYOND SMOOTHIES TO CRAFT WHOLE-FOOD SUPER SHAKES TO ENHANCE NATURAL IMMUNITY, STRENGTH, AND BEAUTY

BY: JOHN SCHOTT

www.SchottsWellness.com

Publishing services provided by 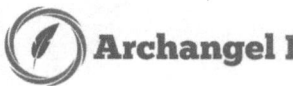 **Archangel Ink**

ISBN: 1517404371
ISBN-13: 978-1517404376

Pristine Hydro images provided by:
PristineHydro Development, Inc.
Ginger Caulkins
24102 El Toro Rd. Ste. D
Laguna Woods, California 92637
(949) 581-9191
livepristine.com

Table of Contents

Introduction

Nutrition Today: A Very Quick Glance

Making sense of the nutrition/health field today can be very overwhelming. I'll take this opportunity to *briefly* share my perspective. The intent is to help plant a seed. I want to offer insights that can help you build a solid foundation to achieve a more vibrant lifestyle.

Most people's approach to health typically begins with a dietary component. It's the most popular. After all, we do have to eat, and tons of books, magazines, and opinions keep on flooding the market. This is where I see an opening to chime in and highlight other areas of the equation. There are overlooked lifestyle aspects that typically suffer at the expense of an excessive focus on food. Diet alone—especially if it's based on a modern or even dogmatic program—is not enough. These days, it is very clear that we have to look at a whole lifestyle approach that involves movement, connecting with nature, and building like-minded communities. There are certain principles that come into play here. For instance, it's critical that we achieve emotional balance and develop stress management strategies for ourselves. It is a main component toward building excellent health. Other elements include finding ways of clearing old traumas and nurturing our nervous system. Smile, laugh, and create effective communication channels in your relationships. These are all pieces of the puzzle. Oh, and don't take yourself or trivial things so seriously. Beyond these, try to be as connected to every element involved in your life. In other words, be present. And of course, this also involves being aware of where our food comes from.

Our environment also plays a key role. The water element is extremely valuable to understand and is greatly underestimated. We will touch upon this subject further in a later section. After all, this is a discourse mostly about liquids. Incorporating fresh and ionized clean air and non-off-gassing paint to reduce as many toxic elements in our homes is also important.

Practice a form of safe, non-extreme exercise or movement practice. This should ideally involve some form of resistance training to preserve or build muscle. Move, move, move. Whether it's walking, rebounding, dancing, or playing with your kids, all these activities enhance the whole body and lymph system. Keep proper cycles of anabolic (building/growing) and catabolic (breaking down/cleansing) processes rotating throughout your life without going to extremes. Also, get grounded, breathe fresh air, and get proper doses of sunny (vitamin) D.

And, of course, eat well! This is where most of us are getting confused (at times fighting each other and ourselves). We're receiving too much information. A lot of times it's contradictory, and when it's all said and done, for many people, the whole thing becomes a reason to drop eating healthy altogether.

So, barring all of that, approach the food element with an air of simplicity. The gist of it is to eat real food. What does that mean? Well, simply begin by discarding anything that comes from a lab. Try your best to avoid genetically modified and factory-farmed foods. Also, stay clear of ingredient lists that nobody except the scientist that put them on the label in the first place can understand. From there, begin to choose beyond overly processed semblances of food. These include things like high fructose corn syrup; hydrogenated and industrialized oils (even vegetable oils); white sugar; bleached, excessively processed white flour; and white homogenized, pasteurized factory-farm dairy. As we consider all those factors, we begin to construct a well-rounded approach to eating, one based somewhat on an ancestral, yet modernized, version of our evolutionary "hunting and gathering" practice. So, to pay tribute to the Paleo folks and raw-food vegans, this is an overall solid starting point. The bulk of our nutrients will come from healthy animal foods and fresh fruits, vegetables, tubers, roots, nuts, seeds, and seaweed. Some dairy, grains, and legumes will come into play here as well. This point is where we tend to veer off into slight layers of complexity, but it shouldn't be too over the top. Furthermore, as we go into the rest of these chapters, I introduce the inclusion of whole liquid meals and drinks into the equation. Here, we explore some elements that incorporate the use of true superfoods, herbs, and wonders of our technological world.

Again, take into account that this is just an introduction to the vast world of nutrition. It's my intent to highlight the use of mindful awareness and see how so many different concepts can fit into the rest of what is involved in these pages, recipes, and techniques. In some areas, there will be considerations as to the type of dairy that may or may not be beneficial. Some people will insist on staying true to their low-carb preferences. Others choose to eternally abstain from the use of any animal product. I get it, and all considerations are respected and honored. There are always ways to tweak and change things up. Taking liberties and having the freedom to build on what's being presented here is actually encouraged. So, take as much as you can from this book. Make it your own or disregard any part that you see fit. In the end, your intuition, experiences, and desires are what matter most. My hope is to create a fun environment, present new ideas, and deliver a unique approach that will enhance the magical genre of smoothies and shakes.

To your health always.

Chapter 1:

Not Another Smoothie Book

Why This Booklet

I know there are so many smoothie, juice, and shake recipe books out in the market today. Not to mention there are endless blogs, web pages, and food-based sites that offer tons of ideas on the topic. My experience with most of these is that they are typically based on a lot of the same principles. Here's the rundown, more or less: You take some milk, apple or orange juice, soy milk, or another inexpensive (and, most of the time, low-quality) ingredient as the base and start there. Then you add a bunch of fruit, maybe some kale, and a sweetener of some sort. Perhaps you feel like adding some nice store-bought yogurt or a powdered green blend with 1,000 ingredients in it. Blend it up and—*boom!*—you have a smoothie. Change a few things up and thousands of recipes follow. Most of the time, there is no strategic approach being followed. At times, smoothies become a thoughtless abyss of sameness.

I'm also aware that there are a few Paleo and raw-food vegan smoothie recipe books available as well. These, to their credit, serve as a great alternative to the mainstream selections. They at least offer upgraded concepts to the other more popular smoothie books. They also go beyond what we see being offered in smoothie bar chains across the country. But, for the most part, by following the bulk of most of those recipes, you're most likely making the same typical fare at home.

So at this point, you may be thinking, "OK, hot Schott, how's your book any different? Here comes yet another smoothie recipe book, prepackaged with a different look and pictures." I'm here to say, as Mr. Wayne Campbell once so eloquently stated, "Not!" All joking aside, in this book I want to offer a true nutritional alternative to making smoothies and shakes. Moreover, I would like to present a systems approach that will help craft whole-food, nutrient-dense liquid meals. The techniques and recipes that follow were put together through many years of trial and success. A lot of the shakes and drinks here come from thousands of shakes I have made throughout the years of successfully running a smoothie bar within the walls of my own organic restaurant.

This booklet represents a strategic tool that can be incorporated into the daily hustle of modern-day living. Let's face it—everyone today is busy. Creating robust health and making nourishing meals, like in the old days, is slightly more challenging than before. There are always ways, however, that we can make our health a top priority. Consequently, unique strategies exist to prepare unbelievably delicious and healthy meals in less than 15 minutes. (That is a subject for another booklet that's in the works.) Making nutrient-dense liquid meals fast and easy is a very helpful way for us to achieve our nutrition goals. The techniques and recipes in this booklet will also teach you how to incorporate cleansing strategies for detoxification. Some of these shakes can help clear the body of excess debris. In this way, we create a pathway to help the body rebuild itself with a higher degree of strength later on. The liquid nutrition approach will also lend itself to introducing medicinal and supplemental foods in an easy-to-digest and very efficient delivery system. So to sum up, the booklet is designed to use technology wisely and efficiently in order to enhance our overall health strategy.

Liquid "Meals": My Approach

The idea of being on liquid foods may seem to quite intimidating for many, but it has some great advantages and rewards. I personally incorporate different cycles, depending on circumstances, time, and activities. There are times when a good percentage of my eating is done by way of a glass or bowl. The addition of this practice is a wonderful art, and one should partake in it as much as desired—not just for cleansing purposes. If this is done correctly by incorporating the right superfoods and constructing nutrient-dense meals composed of enough of the main macronutrients, the experience can be quite rewarding. Also, having proper knowledge of how to correctly use fiber, and where and if the practice of juicing fits (understanding both juices and smoothies, and their roles) is a great plus. Using natural whole fruit, chia seeds, or some coconut, for example, makes a big difference and gets us away from using excessive fiber or powders that hurt us more than help. By adding the techniques and recipes in this book, one can achieve tremendous life-altering levels of nutrition.

A properly assembled super shake, smoothie, elixir, or soup can be a great meal replacement. It can also serve as an additional meal if bulking up, a cleansing drink, an antioxidant and medicinal delivery system, or all of the above. I utilize all these options for different purposes and circumstances. For instance, if I'm doing a semi-intermittent fasting day from dinner to dinner, I may choose to incorporate something that has a bit more spunk rather than a simple glass of water with magnesium. In such a case, I'll do some fresh coconut water or, better yet, a coconut water kefir lemon cocktail (see recipe). This particular drink is rich in enzymes and gut-healing probiotic microorganisms. Sometimes I'll also use an herbal infusion or chaga decoction with some wild honey or stevia drops. This way, I'm really not taking in any calories while doing the fast, but I'm also delivering some electrolytes, minerals, and some form of easy-to-digest herbs and glucose. Another example is regarding what we call breakfast—a lot of times, when I break my overnight fast, I begin my day with a high-quality, exotic fruit protein shake that has elements in it that you will hardly find in other protein shakes in the market (more on this later).

The last thing I want to mention in this section is that I'm a big fan of the concept of pro-youthing, better known as anti-aging. The liquid nutrition approach lends itself very well to achieving high levels of this. For one, it assists in reducing calorie intake while conserving nutrition, if done correctly. And a lot of us are aware that proper use of calorie modification while focusing on nutrient density is a potentially viable anti-aging strategy. I offer a bit of a spin on this, as I believe that a properly planned intermittent fasting program, combined with some of these nutrient-dense drinks, allows for an effective pro-youthing strategy.

Note: *In some of the recipes, I recommend adding certain superfoods and whole-food supplements to your drinks. Some of these additions are not necessarily the tastiest, but there is always a way around it. When adding an unappetizing ingredient—for example, a heavy dose of spirulina to a drink—I usually set aside about 3–5 ounces of my original shake or smoothie in a shot glass. I then add the supplement or superfood to the shot and enjoy the other 12–32 ounces of the drink slowly, savoring every gulp. I get feedback from so many people that they tried so-and-so's recipe and it tasted awful. Typically, this happens when you take a strong-tasting superfood, herb, or other such ingredient, and mix it with the entire smoothie. People are often lured by the nutrient profile of these ingredients, which look great on paper, but don't necessarily translate into a tasty final product. That is why I like this simple tip that makes the experience that much more delightful. It's all a matter of choice, but there are always creative ways to take in everything that is necessary for complete health.*

Chapter 2:

Begin Here

The Prized Element: PristineHydro

We begin with the topic of water because, after all, this is the ingredient we will use the most in this book. All coconut milks, teas, or any of the other starting bases will require good-quality water. This is where we commence the smoothie- and shake-making process. As humans, we are composed of anywhere from 60%–80% water. This is why it is of great importance to use the very best pristine water available.

Today, most water sources are missing vital components, healing properties, and essential elements. The municipal system offers us a cocktail of toxic and damaging ingredients, including fluoride, chlorine, heavy metals, and other constituents. These can all be very counterproductive to one's health strategy. Typically, such sources also have a molecular structure that is incorrect and too large. All these factors make it difficult for the body to achieve proper hydration, and assimilate and transport nutrients through cellular membranes. In the end, it makes the water less miscible with blood. It also makes it more challenging to flush or wash out toxins from the body. Water in plastic bottles that has been sitting on trucks—which is just as devitalized and is potentially filled with xenoestrogens—is not that much better. Drinking and using pristine and high-quality water truly does matter. It makes our super shakes, elixirs, and smoothies stand out. It's almost a shame to dismiss the importance of water when one considers that some of the superfoods and ingredients being recommended here can be pricey. For instance, to mix a shake that has the best-quality colostrum powder with tap water defeats the purpose of trying to make the world's best super shake.

Finding Good-Quality Water

I understand that many of us may have limited ability to obtain great water. Finding a true living spring, even from a great resource like findaspring.com, and actually making time to visit it consistently is, more often than not, a difficult process. I'm a solutions-minded type of individual. When life presents challenges, I dive in to look for the number one, most well-researched answer I can find. So, the great news is that there is an outstanding choice to make our starting star ingredient the most optimal and easily available.

The Prized Element: PristineHydro

After many years of researching water, I came across an incredible solution that offers the highest quality water. It takes ordinary tap water and converts it to pristine, highly structured, oxygenated, sustainable, magnesium bicarbonate-rich, living water from the convenience of your home. It's called PristineHydro, and the system is modeled after the complete hydrological cycle of the planet. If you would like to learn more about this wonderful technology, please visit PristineHydro.com. It is one of the best overall health investments anyone can make. It's the only water system I recommend wholeheartedly. They have under-the-counter, travel, and over-the-counter units that turn municipal water into the best water anyone can drink. The system goes beyond reverse osmosis (RO) and distillation, and it is far better than water ionizers and stale, overly priced bottled waters. Again, check out their site for great videos, comparisons, and further information, and make the most educated decision.

PristineHydro™

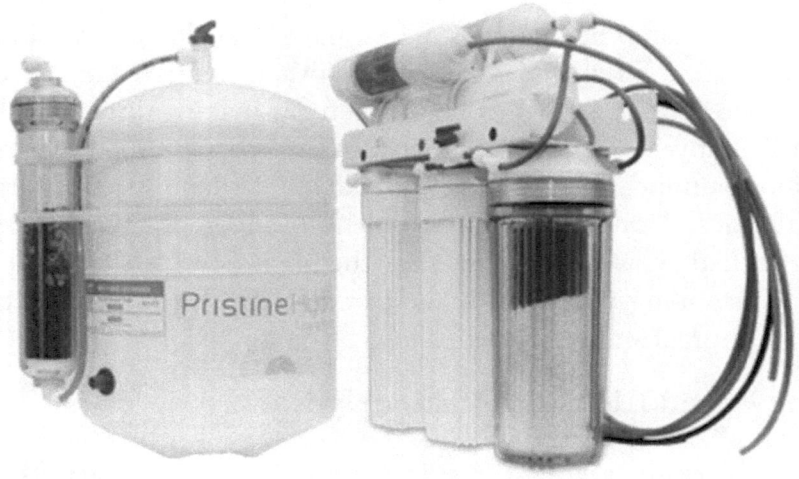

I also understand that some may not have the means and are not quite ready to invest in a PristineHydro water system (I think they do offer payment plans, but I'm not sure how they work). So does that mean these wonderful shakes and smoothies are off the table? Not at all. The idea is to do the best you can where you are. Move in a direction that eventually leads to the highest option available at the moment. What follows are alternative ideas intended to get you started right away.

Like I said, the starting point is to obtain the purest water available. So although in the long run it is not the most sustainable option for the dollar and planet, spring water bottled in glass is a decent option. Brands like Mountain Valley, AquaPanna, and Saratoga Springs are good options. If those aren't within reach, then obtaining bottled distilled water is another option. Unfortunately, to my knowledge, these all come bottled in plastic. After that, you can try other bottled spring water, spring water delivered at home in 5-gallon bottles, or even an inexpensive RO unit. In the end, these will be more expensive long-term.

Note: *If some of the above alternative recommendations are chosen, here are some recommendations for making the water even a little bit better by "charging" it. There are many ways of charging water, and some methods are more complex than others. The simplest way to make whatever water on hand somewhat charged is by, again, starting with the purest water and then throwing a pinch of sun-dried sea salt in it. Next, you spin it with a wooden stick, clockwise, by hand. Other simple things to enhance water include the use of magnets or crystals like quartz and lodestone. Typically, the stones go inside the tank with the water, and magnets wrap around the container that holds the water.*

Chapter 3:

Stock Up and Organize

Optimize Your Kitchen for Success

Equipment and Tools of the Trade

The main piece of equipment in shake mastery is obviously the blender. There are different degrees and types to choose from, but there are four main categories to consider.

The first is the high-investment, top-of-the-line option. Here, we typically have two main choices—Vitamix and Blendtec. These are the highest-priced blenders, ranging from $350 to $500 or more, depending on model, seller, etc. These are definitely an investment that does pay off in the long run. These machines are built well and last long. They are designed to withstand lots of use and are worth the value if homemade smoothies and shakes are staples in your eating program. They also are the best if you plan to use them for other food-making purposes. They're great for sauces, dressings, pates, desserts, soups, and a few other things. My favorite, by far, is Vitamix. I've had mine for more than 10 years, and aside from changing the blade every so often (I use it a lot!), I've never had a problem. I also like Vitamix because, unlike the Blendtec models that are all electric and automated, I can have more manual control of it. Other similar brands with price variances are the Omniblend (~$289) and the Tempest by Hamilton Beach (~$520). I cannot comment on these last two brands since I've had no real need to test them.

The second option would be the hybrid versions of the big boy blenders made as a more inexpensive option. Here, we have models like the Ninja. These are pretty decent. I'm not much of a fan of these because typically, the blade piece is not the most practical of designs. It has good power, however, and will get the job done. Its durability is unknown since they are all relatively new, and I honestly have had no need to put these to any type of test. For $60 to $150, it can be a more doable investment. Other similar brands are the Versa by Oster ($200+) and Omega (~$170).

The third option is the NutriBullet option. This is pretty much the only option in this category. I'm not one to endorse a product without other alternatives, but for a simple and very effective tool for making single-serve smoothies and shakes, this is a very good gadget. It's also great for traveling. It really does blend in a way that is smooth, extracts elements from the food appropriately, and is convenient. The price is decent as well—most go for about $100. Again, this is in a category of its own because it's not up to par with one of the more heavy-duty blenders, but it is also a notch above the conventional household blender, which is in our last category.

The final category houses the good old blender that most of us were raised with—the ones that have paved the way to the more evolved models mentioned above. These should not be dismissed, however, since any smoothie or shake in this book can be made using any of these models. Typically, they range from $35 to $250. The higher end of this range is what constitutes the more professional version of this type of blender. The brands typically found in this category are Hamilton Beach, Black & Decker, Calphalon, KitchenAid, and Cuisinart.

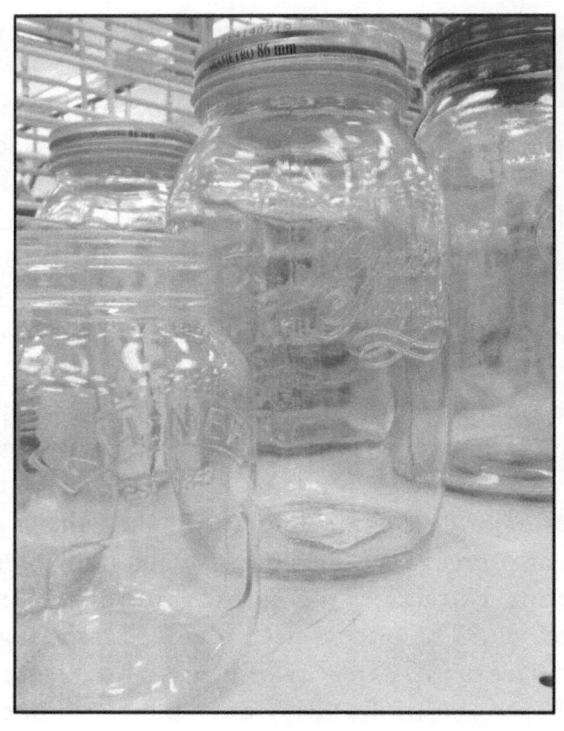

Besides a good blender, there is not much more equipment necessary to make shakes. It's good, however, to invest in a few measuring spoons, a good 1-gallon pitcher (this one is to store nut milk), a good knife, and a good number of different sizes of mason jars. The mason jars are pretty essential. These not only serve as a cool glass or mug but, to me, are essential for storing ingredients. From cacao powder to whey, lucuma, chia, goji berries, and other herbs and medicinal mushrooms, these jars are great for keeping the kitchen organized. They also help make the alchemist in you come alive since you can get inspired when you open your cupboards or look at your shelves. Moreover, these clear jars help keep easy inventory since you can actually see when ingredients are running low. If you like hot drinks, these can also be used if you purchase a cool sleeve from Cuppow or Surthrival. Mason jars come in many sizes that offer different uses. They have 16-ounce jars for individual shakes, 32-ounce jars for a bigger meal replacement or a quart of milk. Also, there are 64-

ounce jars to use for half-gallon portions of nut milk and herbal infusions.

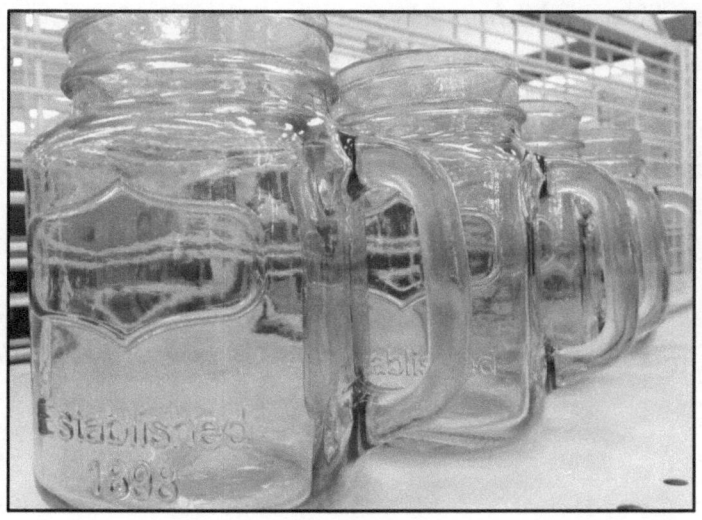

One final note and consideration to best succeed in mastering shakes is to get organized in general. This may be obvious, and a lot of the considerations stated previously assist with that. However, make a point to open up space in your cupboards, in the freezer, and on the counter. Take note of things in your kitchen that haven't been used in a while. Replace those with the new things now being discovered. Lastly, spend a few minutes analyzing your space, so that you can establish a flow. Today, there are always time constraints with everything we do, and optimizing flow in your kitchen can save you time, make your process more efficient, and, in the end, can help deliver even better results. This can look like simply placing your jars on a shelf next to the blender (at least the ones that you come back to use time and time again). There will be some bulk ingredients that you know are your staples that will require other storage strategies, but you get the idea. Have fun in the kitchen.

Note: *Investing in a good-quality slow cooker is also one of my highest recommendations. It's one of my favorites and it's a go-to tool in the kitchen. It makes life easy and efficient. You may be saying, "Why the heck is a slow cooker being mentioned in a shake book?" This handy piece of equipment is useful not only for roasts, veggies, and pull-the-meat-off-the-bone dishes, but it's fantastic for making decoctions of tough herbs and medicinal mushrooms. For example, you can place some chaga in the slower cooker with pristine water, turn the slow cooker on low, and leave it for hours, extracting some of the mushroom's medicine. You can use the liquid for tea bases and soups. Speaking of soups, using the slow cooker is a convenient and great way to make collagen- and mineral-rich broth. These also come into play in this book since I offer some soup recipes and ideas in addition to the smoothies and shakes.*

Chapter 4:

The Only Base Worth Using

Wild Milk: No Store-Bought Milk Here

Firstborn, here's a full and honest disclosure:

This is the part in the book where I introduce a product that I have developed and sell. I know you may be thinking, "I didn't buy this book in order to be sold anything extra." Or worse, "This guy has written a shake book so that he can promote and sell a product to be used with his recipes." To be honest, there is some truth to that. The Wild Milk product was created for nutritional benefit, efficiency, and as an alternative to store-bought milks. Aside from this, there isn't anything in the market that doesn't have gut-irritating ingredients. Also, making nut milks from scratch is not practical for most people. Heck, I started using this special concentrate in my business precisely because it's more efficient for me to use when making my delicious nutrient-dense shakes. Purchasing bulk amounts of the typical boxed milk was never an option for me. Anyway, this specific book was definitely *not* created with the purpose of selling Wild Milk. Again, I understand skepticism, especially in a growing health field that touts miracle "solutions" each day. Like most, I understand the endless sea of sales pitches we face with an overabundance of products now available. I too have seen a lot of products in the organic market being heavily promoted to do exactly those things. Most of the time, they're actually quite disappointing, the value of what you purchase is subpar, and it delivers only empty promises. So, considering all of the above, the last thing I want to do is to be another pusher of yet another product. Or worse, to potentially base an entire educational tool on some fully capitalist-minded agenda. It's not my intent to do that. The last thing I want to do is make anyone dependent on any one thing. I include it here because I really like and use my own product. I truly believe it to be an innovative alternative and the best shake/smoothie base around. It's also very cool for storage and travel purposes. I sometimes store up to 20 gallons of Wild Milk in my cupboard. There is, however, no need to buy it. This is why, in the next sections, I will actually give you insights on how to make your own and all the techniques necessary for you to create and use other base options. And yes, if you truly feel there is absolutely no choice right now other than going to a store to buy a boxed almond milk, then that's fine too. The idea behind this book is to add new ingredients, techniques, concepts, and value. Sometimes the stress of having to make something from scratch is not worth a little bit of guar gum, carrageenan, or any of the other common stabilizers and thickeners in commercial products. Always do the best you can. One last note—aside from perhaps using Wild Milk, there are other ingredients listed here that require additional purchases, of course. Let's face it—we live in a commercially driven world. There are rare scenarios where you get the opportunity to go outside your door, milk your own cow or goat and use its surplus colostrum, heavy cream, and yogurt, and pick wild berries from the field next door. So yes, I will be adding links to the highest quality superfoods, protein powders, and some wild fruit sources.

Milk Alternatives

So, if you don't want to buy Wild Milk, no problem. Here's the scoop on alternatives:

A) Canned Coconut Milk

A good-quality, full-fat, organic canned coconut milk can serve as a great starting point to a shake or smoothie. The trick is to know how to use it. So, if a shake calls for 1½ cups (12 ounces) of starter base, what I typically suggest is to use ¼ to ½ cup of the canned coconut milk and the remainder in pristine water. This will give you a full-bodied consistency and also help cut down on an excess amount of calories. Of course, feel free to use more of the coconut milk if desired. Just know that there is more fat and calories with that option, and the shake will definitely be richer. If you're trying to gain weight or build up your body, this is actually an interesting strategy to explore. On the other hand, if you're trying to lose some weight, adding a bit more coconut milk and using the shake as a meal replacement can also be something to consider. If there is a concern with the can's materials leaching into the food, then explore other options, or at least find the BPA-free options. I personally don't get too concerned with that detail since I use the canned coconut milks only once in a while. I also use near-infrared saunas to sweat toxins out and practice other detox principles regularly.

B) Instant Nut and Seed Milks

This section is where innovation meets ancestral approaches. To make an instant nut milk, it is as simple as taking some nut or seed butter and blending it with water. That's it! It doesn't get any easier than that. The trick is to have correct proportions so that the nut milk is not watered down or too concentrated. The smoothie has the potential to feel too heavy or like something is missing if the proportions aren't right. The other factor is to include a living sea salt when making instant nut milk. A pinch for a cup of milk will typically suffice. This little trick will make the whole thing round off the recipe or come together. So to get a little technical, typically about 1 heaping tablespoon of nut or seed butter will create the right consistency for 1 cup of milk. This, paired with a pinch of salt, will get you the full effect. You can pre-blend this and add smoothie ingredients later or place all ingredients in at once—both work. So feel free to use almond butter, sunflower seed butter, or even coconut butter for all these instant milk options.

I have also used Irish moss many times to enhance the full-bodied effects of nut milks. Irish moss is a seaweed that, when processed properly, has a very subtle to nonexistent flavor. I like to incorporate it into my bases or shakes from time to time because it adds nutritional value, mucilaginous components that can assist with a healthy gut, and makes for a thicker and fuller experience without having to add more fat. Now, I'm very aware that Irish moss is also known as carrageenan. This is important to recognize because, after all, carrageenan is ironically one of the added ingredients in boxed milks that can irritate the gut and possibly create health challenges. I have seen research on carrageenan, which is one of the reasons I don't use boxed milks. Bearing all that in mind, the process I use with a raw Irish moss is actually quite different. In this context, I believe Irish moss can be beneficial, and I have no qualms with its use. I have never had a negative reaction with Irish moss when used in its whole-food state. I will share the process and steps as to how to prepare Irish moss at the end of this section. It is more work, so keep that in mind.

I also want to mention that utilizing really fresh and high-quality hemp seeds can work with the instant milk technique. I am personally not a fan of this option because hemp, in my perspective and research, is still a relatively new experimental food. There are questions as to the possibility that hemp as a food can have high concentrations of estrogen similar to soy and flax. For this main reason, I typically stay away from it. Awhile back, I switched over to making all my bases from fresh hemp seeds. My impression was that I felt my libido and overall drive drop significantly. Was it due to excessive estrogen and hormonal changes? The truth is that it's difficult to prove, but that's my theory and the feeling at the moment. So, with all that to consider, my suggestion is to proceed mindfully with all hemp products. Also, hemp is highly concentrated in omega-3 fatty acids. These tend to get rancid fairly quickly, especially if exposed to excessive heat, light, and long-term storage. This is why if you've ever experimented with making hemp milk and the flavor is bitter and strong, it is typically due to rancid seeds—not something I recommend. Rancid fat is rancid fat, no matter its nutritional profile and potential benefits.

The final option in this section is using unsweetened shredded coconut as a base. Shredded coconut is a great option because it's quite easy to use and fairly inexpensive. The trick is to take about ½ to 1 cup of coconut shreds and blend at high speed with 1 to 1½ cups pristine water. Once blended you can simply strain, add a pinch of salt, and use as your base. I also like to add 1 to 2 tablespoons of coconut oil to this since the dry shredded coconut is usually missing the full fatty consistency desired for a nice buttery type of nut milk.

> **Note**: *With any of these recipes, feel free to add a little bit of wildflower raw honey, grade B maple syrup, palm sugar, or liquid stevia to add an extra touch of sweetness.*

Check out Chapter 7, where I share my approach in further detail and recipes to make both instant nut milks and nut milks made from scratch for those who still love the process of making a more involved nut milk.

C) Using Herbs

Using herbs as a base can be tricky. A lot of elixir or medicinal shakes typically begin with these options. Although I think it's great to include these, I also personally like a richer consistency as my starting point. The great news is that the instant nut milk strategy can be easily incorporated by mixing the nut butters and salt with the tea base instead of just water. Some of the most popular herbs I like using are gynostemma, chaga, nettle leaf, and sometimes even yerba mate if I prefer a more earthy flavor. All these are a matter of preference and ideas to play with. Just remember, when working with herbs—especially on a daily basis—it's best to choose the adaptogenic and tonic herbs. Tonic herbs are typically those that are used to enhance body function in a slow and gentle long-term manner. They are safer to use daily as opposed to stronger, more medicinal herbs that are more concentrated and typically used for a specific purpose. The main way to use herbs in a base is to have an infusion or decoction already premade.

D) Using Dairy

Using dairy is both a tricky and sensitive topic. After all, we should consider that factory-farmed, pasteurized, homogenized, and non-organic milk from confined operations can be a major piece to our modern-day health challenges. These are typically loaded with antibiotics and other unnatural elements that have been linked to excessive inflammatory and allergenic conditions. However, we do have somewhat of a significant history of using the right type of dairy as a nutritive substance. I am not going to get into a political or ethical debate in this book. Considering all those factors, dairy has to be something that at the very least is presented as a possible base option for a shake or smoothie. The one thing that I will recommend is that if using this as an option, it is best to attempt to access the highest quality dairy you can get. This typically looks like a 100% grass-fed, organic, and, ideally, raw option. Also consider whether your family lineage has a successful history of using dairy. That and possibly an elimination diet for a short period of time with the reintroduction of dairy can give you a solid clue as to whether this food works in your favor.

E) Other Base Ideas

Many times people choose other more common bases such as coconut water, apple, pineapple, orange, or even cold-pressed juice. Although all of these can work as a base, I personally don't like them or use them. Perhaps for a fruit smoothie, these can work fine in terms of flavor. When looking for a super shake or milkshake consistency, however, these really miss the mark. Besides all that, working with juice as a base is something I recommend doing only sparingly. Remember, all these are very concentrated forms of sugar–natural sugar, but sugar nonetheless. I am not in the camp that believes all sugar is bad or that low-carb is the answer to all health challenges, but at the same time, depending on metabolism, circumstances, and activity levels, pure fruit juice—even cold-pressed—may not be the best route to take for many.

Chapter 5:

What is a Superfood?

Superfoods Worth Using

S uperfoods. This word, like so many others in the health field, is like a loaded gun. It's ready to fire into a wide-open and vulnerable audience that is starving for the next quick fix and instant-gratification solution. From bulletproof coffee to goji berries, moringa, kale, and God knows what else, *superfoods* is a term that, at the very least, deserves some further exploration.

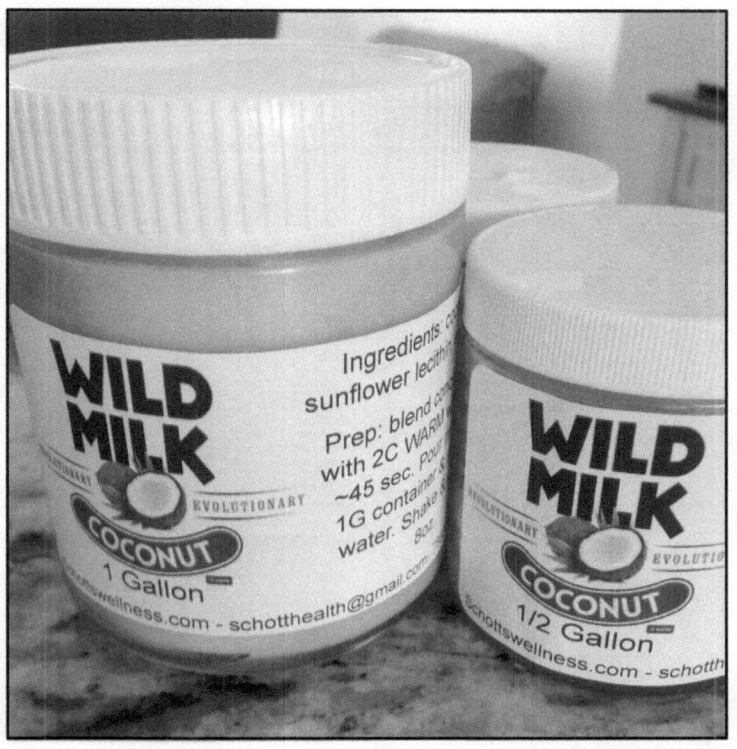

So, what is a superfood? It is a food considered to be very beneficial for one's health. It is a food with a wide spectrum of nutrients that is power-packed with higher concentrations of constituents touted superior to regular food. So, of course, with such claims of superiority, the next step is to bring in the heavy marketing and make some money. After all, as long as there is a newer, better model of superfoods coming off the lot, more sales can be generated. So what once began with a lonely blue-green algae (spirulina) has now escalated into a laundry list of "magical" foods promising the ever-coveted fountain of youth. Take the following label of a popular superfood product as an example, and you get an idea of what we're dealing with:

Supplement Facts

Serving Size: 1 scoop (42 g)   Servings Per Container: 30

	Amount Per Serving	% Daily Value**
Calories	160	
Calories from Fat	10	
Total Fat	1 g	2%
Saturated Fat	0 g	
Trans Fat	0 g	
Cholesterol	0 mg	0%
Sodium	70 mg	3%
Total Carbohydrate	20 g	7%
Dietary Fiber	4 g	16%
Sugars	10 g	
Protein	15 g	30%

PROPRIETARY VEGAN PROTEIN BLEND: 19 g †
Raw sprouted whole grain brown rice protein, Sacha inchi (*Plukenetia volubilis*, seed).

PROPRIETARY SUPERFOOD / FIBER BLEND: 8,350 mg †
Coconut flower nectar, Sprouted Chia (*Salvia hispanica*, seed), Sprouted Flax (*Linum usitatissimum*, seed), Pea fiber (*Pisum spp.*, seed), Quinoa (*Chenopodium quinoa*, seed), Amaranth (*Amaranthus hypochondriacus*, seed).

PROPRIETARY ADAPTOGEN HERB BLEND: 1,675 mg †
Maca root (*Lepidium meyenii*), Astragalus root (*Astragalus membranaceus*), Ashwagandha root (*Withania somnifera*), Maitake mushroom (*Grifola frondosa*), Cordyceps (*Cordyceps sinensis*, fungi), Reishi mushroom (*Ganoderma lucidum*), Holy basil (*Ocimum sanctum*, leaf), Schisandra (*Schisandra spp.*, fruit), Ginkgo (*Ginkgo biloba*, leaf).

	Amount Per Serving	% Daily Value**
ANTIOXIDANT / SUPER-FRUIT BLEND:	1,400 mg	†

Pomegranate (*Punica granatum*, fruit), Acerola cherry (*Malpighia glabra*, fruit), Bilberry (*Vaccinium sp.*, fruit), Goji berry (*Lycium barbarum*), Camu-Camu (*Myrciaria dubia*, fruit), Açaí (*Euterpe oleracea*, fruit), Blueberry (*Vaccinium angustifolium*, fruit), Citrus bioflavonoids, Green tea (*Camellia sinensis*, leaf), Rose hips (*Rosa canina*, fruit).

PROPRIETARY FRUIT POWDER BLEND: 1,300 mg †
Strawberry (*Fragaria chiloensis*, berry), Apple pectin (*Malus pumila*, fruit), Banana (*Musa spp.*, fruit), Pineapple (*Ananas comosus*, fruit), Papaya (*Carica papaya*, fruit).

PROPRIETARY PREBIOTIC AND PROBIOTIC BLEND: 1,075 mg †
Yacon root (*Smallanthus sonchifolius*), Lactobacillus sporogenes (as Bacillus coagulans) naturally micro-encapsulated.

PHYTONUTRIENT / SUPER-GREENS BLEND: 750 mg †
Spirulina (*Arthrospira platensis*, *Arthrospira maxima*, whole), Chlorella (*Chlorella sp.*, whole), Spinach (*Spinacia oleracea*, leaf), Barley grass (*Hordeum vulgare*), Kamut grass (*Triticum turanicum*), Oat grass (*Avena sativa*), Wheat grass (*Triticum aestivum*).

MSM (Methylsulfonylmethane) 250 mg †

PROPRIETARY DIGESTIVE ENZYME BLEND: 100 mg †
Protease, Amylase, Cellulase, Lipase, Papain, Lactase, Bromelain.

**Percent Daily Values are based on a 2,000-calorie diet.
†Daily Value not established.

OTHER INGREDIENTS: Tapioca, Natural flavors (strawberry, banana, pineapple), Konjac gum, Beet juice powder, Citric acid, Natural sweetener (proprietary blend of erythritol, oligosaccharides and natural flavors), Cinnamon powder, Himalayan salt, Stevia, and Luo han guo fruit.

ALLERGY INFORMATION: This product is manufactured in a plant that also processes soy, egg, fish, crustacean shellfish, tree nuts, and wheat (gluten) ingredients.

STORAGE: Store in a cool, dry place. To ensure freshness, consume within 4 to 5 weeks of opening.

WARNING: Consult with a healthcare professional if you are pregnant, breast feeding, or if you have any medical conditions. Keep out of reach of children.

Amino Acid Profile***

Amino Acid	Amount Per Serving	Amino Acid	Amount Per Serving	Amino Acid	Amount Per Serving	Amino Acid	Amount Per Serving
Alanine	850 mg	Glycine	699 mg	Methionine‡	398 mg	Tryptophan‡	192 mg
Arginine	1,261 mg	Histidine‡	364 mg	Phenylalanine‡	871 mg	Tyrosine	784 mg
Aspartic Acid	1,398 mg	Isoleucine‡	658 mg	Proline	734 mg	Valine‡	926 mg
Cystine	287 mg	Leucine‡	1,322 mg	Serine	791 mg		
Glutamic Acid	2,874 mg	Lysine‡	406 mg	Threonine‡	565 mg		

***Typical amount in bio-fermented raw sprouted whole-grain brown rice protein found in Shakeology.
‡Essential Amino Acids.

On paper, the product looks promising and quite possibly amazing. In reality, however, when common sense rears its "ugly" head and the hype wears off, we suddenly realize that we're left with a questionable idea at best. Out of all the magical ingredients listed, perhaps some deliver on what is being claimed. Moreover, with so many ingredients crammed into one formula, it's less likely that the amount of each ingredient is enough to make a difference. And even if the quantity was available, the price would be astronomical. Finally, the excessive amount of ingredients together will probably make it difficult to properly digest and process efficiently inside the body. At this point, what I personally advocate is to invest in quality, the right quantity, and overall value of your ingredients. I also look at these foods from the angle of traditional and longest historical use. As you will notice, I also feel that with technology there is the potential to discover new methods of using "older" foods that we previously had not been able to successfully harvest: new foods like marine phytoplankton and a small number of potentially healing seed oils, that, if extracted properly and with the right precision, can present positive real-food alternatives.

So what follows is my condensed list of what I consider a traditional, yet technological and modern approach, to nutrient-dense foods. Many of these we've been using for a very long time in different forms and using diverse delivery systems. All of these can actually offer some incredible nutritional benefits. Call them superfoods or what you will, I use them in my shakes because they present us with a lot of value. Consequently, and I have to be honest here, as of now I don't feel one can build a complete diet based on superfoods alone. Just because they are potentially "the most nutrient-dense foods on the planet," there are still other elements that must be included to fully tailor our eating strategy. I personally tried to fully live on superfoods at one point, and without a balanced whole-food program, I ran into deficiencies. I simply wasn't getting the results I wanted or making the most optimal choice for my health. In hindsight, if I wasn't experimenting with my ever-evolving super shake approach being shared here, I possibly could have done even more damage to my own health than I did. As such, these shakes were potentially my saving grace from getting into a much deeper point of no return.

Here's a list of what I have used in the past. Beyond those, what follows are the ones I now recommend and expand upon.

- baobab
- camu camu
- acai
- ashwaganda
- tribulus
- moringa
- green tea
- rhodiola
- maqui
- hemp
- golden berries
- durian
- noni
- schizandra
- mangosteen
- diverse green powder blends, including sprout powders
- astragalus
- mucuna
- ginseng
- various special juice concentrates
- other Ayurvedic extracts and more

The following list has a somewhat in-depth look into what I now use more consistently. These, at times, I use as staples, and I rotate most of them in and out of my diet:

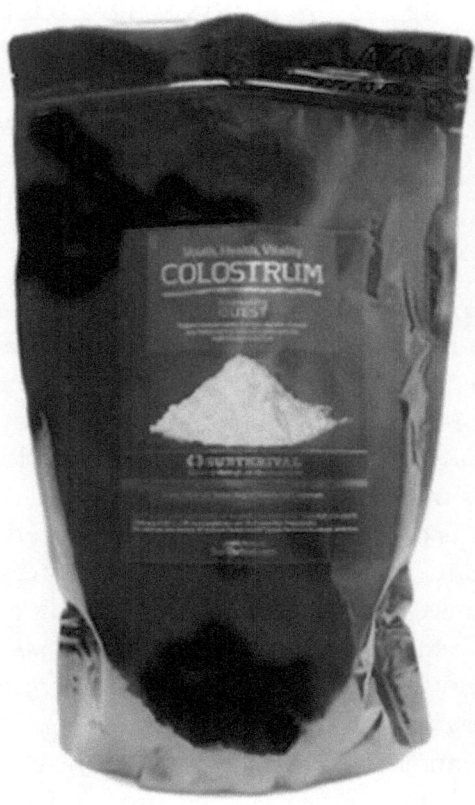

Colostrum - All mammals' first and most complete food. It has an entire complex of nutrients and immune growth factors (IGF1) that build and rebuild your immune system from the ground up. It has gut-healing constituents, assists in fighting against opportunistic microorganisms, and regenerates all body tissues. The colostrum that I recommend here is one that not only represents the highest quality but also adheres to the most sustainable practices. It is true six-hour colostrum, and not a mix of colostrum with transitional milk. It comes from a surplus of the raw material where nothing is taken away from the original species or in an unconscious fashion. Colostrum is the ultimate superfood, and, in my view, a super shake is not complete without it.

Grass-Fed, Low-Temperature, Whole-Whey Protein - It's an extracted protein from a grass-fed, free-roaming, healthy ruminant. It's a fortifying food. In a sense, it is a somewhat singled-out ingredient as it is one of the protein components derived from milk. It serves, however, as a whole element of extreme bioavailable value and a concentrated form of digestible protein. Good-quality whey has been shown in some cases to be cancer preventive and has constituents that create a youthful and regenerative quality. It has the correct and highly available forms of amino acids that potentially create a glutathione surplus. This is a highly valued ideal since glutathione is an extremely important component of robust cellular function. The whey I recommend is not only grass-fed, but it is whole and truly low-temperature extracted. This makes a big difference since the active and beneficial aspects of the whole whey are preserved fully. For years I have tested and researched plant-based protein powders, and none have come close to delivering the building, recovery, and full nutritional benefits of whey. *But John, have you tried pea protein? Or quinoa protein? Or the wonderful complete combinations that new organic companies offer with rice, pea, and hemp proteins properly mixed?* Yes, I have tried and studied them all, and still, none compare. I do use a pumpkin seed and sunflower seed protein from time to time, and if I had to make a vegan choice, these would be the ones I would use. But in the end, nothing comes close to this type of grass-fed, low-temperature, whole whey. See the resources for my top pick and other recommendations.

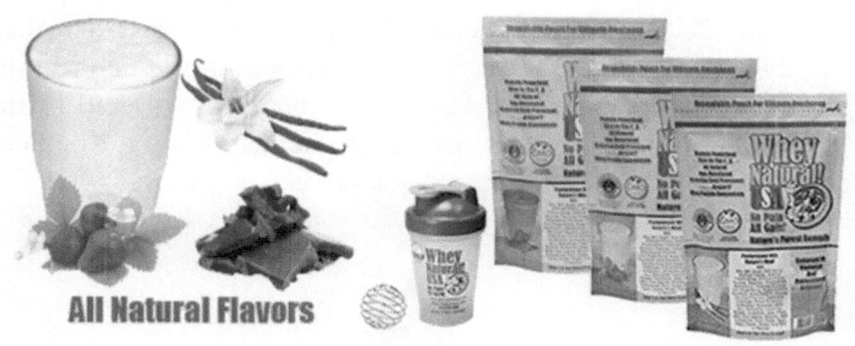

All Natural Flavors

Marine Phytoplankton and Blue-Green Algae

Oceans Alive - Marine phytoplankton is the suspended living seed of the ocean. Here we possibly have the most compatible strand to human DNA from a plant source (*Nannochloropsis gaditana*) that has been properly extracted via sustainable technological means. It's pure energy in a bottle. It feeds your mitochondria directly and enhances neurotransmitter activity. I like this substance because it represents an incredible pro-youthing, cell-nourishing benefit that is quickly making its way as one of the premier foods of the future.

E3 Live - Klamath lake blue-green algae is one of the world's most complete foods. It's a blood cleansing, pro-youthing, brain enhancing, and antioxidant-rich superfood. It's superior to wheatgrass in that it's easier to digest and assimilate, and has way more chlorophyll. Its biochemistry is somewhat different than phytoplankton, and this is why I use them both.

Bee Products - Bee products have a very long history of human consumption. The benefits of royal jelly, bee pollen, propolis, and wild honey are immense. They have been revered by cultures for thousands of years. (See the next chapter on Antidote for a more elaborate description on these.)

Cacao (real chocolate) – it's a nut treasured for its high antioxidant potential, magnesium, and chromium richness, and it has also been used historically as a sacred food and as an herbal medicinal delivery system. As a complete, pure substance, it has an ability to provide energy and enhance mood and brain function. It's best used from a properly handled, cultured form. Check the resource pages for my recommendation on the highest quality cacao products. This substance, like anything, is not for everyone, so be cautious if sensitivities are felt when ingesting.

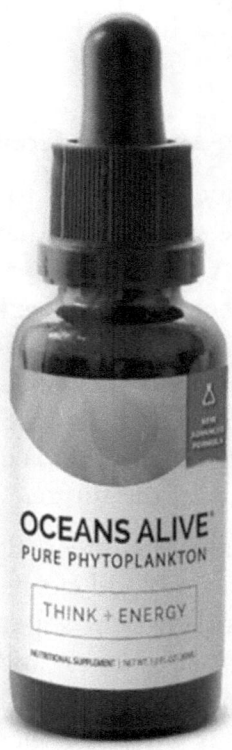

Medicinal Mushrooms - There are numerous medicinal mushrooms available on the market today. Medicinal mushrooms represent a kingdom of both functional food and a branch of tonic herbalism that offers incredible benefits. A medicinal mushroom contains the fruiting body or mycelium of fungi, offering a vast array of polysaccharides like beta-glucans and nutrients like glycoproteins, antioxidants, flavonoids, and tri-terpenes. All these elements make for a food extract that helps modulate the immune system, possibly assists in fighting cancer, and builds incredible amounts of overall strength for the body. There is incredible research behind these, and many good books have been written on the subject. In the resource section, I have listed some of the websites and texts that I recommend if you desire to explore further. For now, my intent is to present an introduction to these worthwhile investments, where to get them, and how to use them. They truly do offer an opportunity to improve health tremendously. My favorite medicinal mushroom is cordyceps. This particular mushroom is well-known to fortify the immune system, build stamina and strength, and also help balance adrenal function and hormones. Several of the more popular, and also quite valuable, medicinal mushrooms are chaga, reishi, *Agaricus blazei* aka the "sun mushroom", maiitake, and shiitake. My recommendation is to begin with one or two and explore which ones you resonate with most. Also, a little further research on each of these can help you determine which one is best to incorporate based on your lifestyle, dietary preferences, and overall needs.

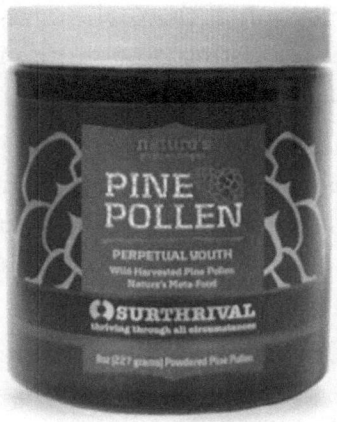

Pine Pollen - As the term states, it is the pollen dropped by the male catkins of the pine tree. It is superior endocrine- and immune-system nourishment. Pine pollen helps to naturally balance the hormonal system with a whole-food, androgen-building complex, immune growth factors, and a complete complex of amino acids. It is the highest whole-food source of natural whole testosterone. It helps to rebuild the body, acts as a youthening agent, and gives you energy to boot.

Additional Powders and Elements to Rotate

Goji Berry – This is a low-glycemic berry that acts as a powerful food to enhance immunity. It is rich in antioxidants and can assist with vision. It's also an overall body tonic and has been used in China as an herb to address a varied amount of body ailments.

Maca – This is a Peruvian root that is a powerful endocrine-strengthening substance. It assists both men and women to nourish libido, energy, and vitality naturally.

Spirulina – This is a blue-green micro algae used throughout history as a whole-body, cellular-rebuilding food. It has three to four times more chlorophyll than wheatgrass, a full complex of amino acids, immune boosting phytonutrients, antioxidants, and is an overall survival food.

Chlorella – Similar to spirulina in all of its benefits, chlorella has the added bonus of chlorella growth factor, which can rebuild your nucleic acid complex, and thus your DNA. It is more cleansing than spirulina since it can go after heavy metals and chemicals. This is a green algae.

Coconut oil – One of nature's best sources of saturated fat, it helps to rebuild hormonal function. It has powerful antimicrobial, anti-fungal, and antiviral properties. It's an instant energizer as it has MCT-type fats that bypass the liver for direct fat-burning access. It helps satiate the appetite and thus helps in weight management.

Mesquite – Mesquite is not considered a 100% superfood, but it delivers unusual amino acids that other foods don't have. It comes from a pod that is rich in calcium, potassium, and other trace elements. It's great in a shake and has a wonderful semisweet, smoky flavor.

Chia – This is a mucilaginous seed that absorbs 4 to 10 times its weight in water, thus helping to keep the body hydrated. It has the closest ratio of omega-3 to omega-6. Chia assists in colon health to rebuild and strengthen body tissues, and it's also a great type of protein. One of the most consistent and effective ways to use chia is to have some hydrated "gel" in the fridge to throw instantly into shakes for nutritional benefits and thickness. The ratio is typically 1 part chia to about 8–12 parts water or nut milk (e.g., 1 tablespoon chia to 8–12 tablespoons water). Of course, making chia porridges is fantastic as well.

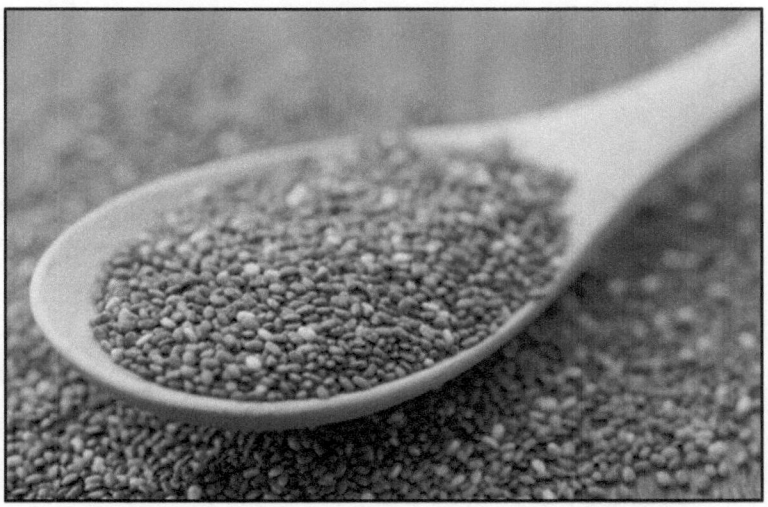

Lucuma – This is powdered eggfruit. It is an excellent source of low-glycemic carbohydrate, fiber, vitamins, and minerals, including remarkable concentrations of beta-carotene, niacin, and iron. Also assists in emulsifying fat.

Tocotrienols – This is uncooked rice bran, a whole-food complex strategically extracted with an activated/timed enzymatic process to bring forth nature's highest source of vitamin E (tocopherols). It is also rich in B vitamins, as well as vitamin A for supreme cardiovascular, neural, and antioxidant ability. It strengthens cell membranes, capillaries, myelin sheathing of nerves, and improves reproductive health.

Irish Moss – One of nature's most incredible wild foods, it is a sea vegetable that offers high-grade nutritional value since it has 92 trace minerals. These can play a key role in activating enzyme and metabolic processes within the body. It can aid in digestion and assimilation of nutrients. It contains hormone-balancing properties, and it's a great weight-loss substance. It has mucilaginous properties, which assist in keeping the GI tract clear of debris and food transit time moving appropriately.

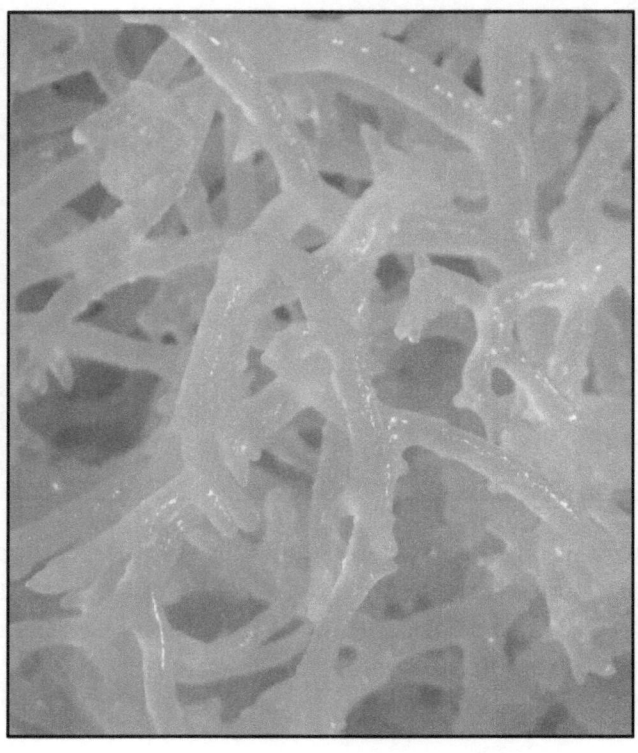

To prepare Irish moss, one must first rinse it well in a strainer and make sure all debris and dirt is washed away. The second step is to soak it overnight in order to allow it to expand and rehydrate. As it plumps up, hidden debris will surface, and one should go strand-by-strand to remove these bits of debris or dirt. Following that, one should re-soak the Irish moss for few minutes in warm to hot water so that it begins to soften, making it easier to blend. Finally, one blends about 3 cups of Irish moss with 2½ cups of warm to hot water. If not using a Vitamix-type blender, use the same ratio with lower quantities. If a thicker consistency is desired, then less water can be mixed. After it's been processed, it lasts in the fridge for a month or so.

Chapter 6:

Antidote

Superfood that Stands Alone

What is Antidote?

Antidote is the most unique superfood-elixir blend. The recipe and idea was created by Glen Caulkins from Pristine Wellness. The main reason it has a whole section here is simple. As the name says it, Antidote is designed to be a potential puzzle piece to the nutritional challenges of the day. In a world where the soil hasn't been properly nurtured and is depleted of essential minerals, and where highly unnatural environments have been created, there is a massive need for special, concentrated foods. The components of these time-tested longevity foods blended together make for a serum that brings forth some of these missing elements. Royal jelly, bee pollen, propolis, grass-fed ghee, coconut oil, shilajit, and wild honey are the main components in the formula. They work synergistically with the right type and concentration of minerals, the highest quality fat to deliver its constituents, and an ample supply of enzymes and healing properties from the bee products. I will further elaborate on the major benefits of these foods specifically toward the end of this section. Before that, I want to state that the mixture definitely has a strong flavor. It's not for everyone. In all honesty, it is not absolutely necessary to use it in a shake or smoothie. Actually, most of the time, I don't use it in this way. I think, any way it is consumed, it's an important component of a successful overall strategy for optimal health. That's why I feel it needs to be included in this book. So the way I personally take it is simple: straight up. I typically eat 1 to 2 tablespoons as medicine almost every day. However, there are also ways to integrate it into a shake.

Antidote Shakes

The best way to use the strong-tasting Antidote serum in a shake is to mask its flavors with strong animal by-product ingredients. Therefore, the base that typically works best (if you have no negative reactions to dairy) will typically be raw, grass-fed cow's or goat's milk. In addition, it's a great idea to also add some farm-fresh yogurt and a little extra honey. Typically, in this blend, use 2 to 4 heaping tablespoons of Antidote. This will be sufficient for a single 16-ounce serving. Another way to experiment is to make bigger batches at a time by doubling or tripling the amount. In this way, you can even use the super shake as a few meal replacements throughout the day until dinner. There are, of course, no rules here. I have used coconut milk and my coconut Wild Milk with Antidote as well, and it works. Here are two examples of Antidote shakes. They can always be tweaked as desired.

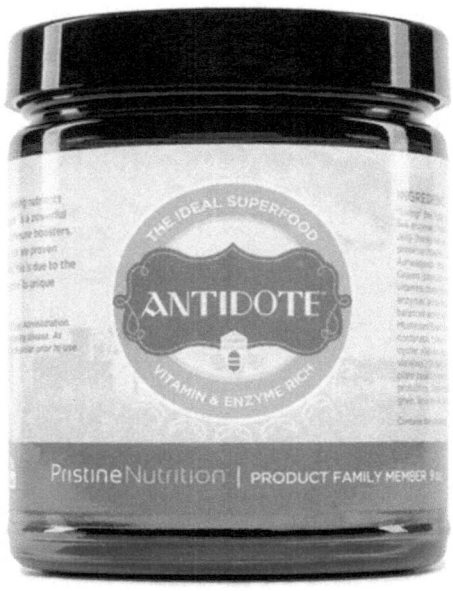

Antidote Basic Shake*

Makes 1 (16-ounce) serving

- ½–1 cup grass-fed raw milk
- ½ cup grass-fed raw yogurt
- 2–4 tablespoons Antidote
- 1–2 tablespoons wild honey
- ½ cup ice or frozen berries
- Blend all ingredients well and enjoy.

*Additions of 1–2 tablespoons colostrum and/or grass-fed, whole-whey protein are recommended as well.

Tropical Chocolate-dote

Makes 1 (16-ounce) serving

- 1 cup Wild Milk, coconut milk, or almond milk
- ½ cup frozen papaya or mamey, if available
- 2–4 tablespoons Antidote
- 1–2 tablespoons cacao powder
- 1 tablespoon cacao nibs
- 1–2 tablespoons colostrum
- 1–2 tablespoons palm sugar or wild honey
- ½ cup ice
- 1–2 tablespoons grass-fed, whole-whey protein (optional)
- Blend all ingredients well and enjoy.

More on What Makes Antidote So Special. . .

Royal Jelly - Royal jelly is a highly nutritious substance created by the worker bees from pollen. It's the exclusive nourishment of the queen bee in the hive. It has a high potential for natural hormone development. It's rich in vitamins, minerals, amino acids, antioxidants, and other elements that fortify cellular function. In this manner, it also fortifies the body with vitality, extra potential energy, and overall strength. It assists in improving mental function, the immune system, and glandular system. It's been studied and found to be high in pantothenic acid, which is the key element in the queen bee's impressive longevity and fertility. There are numerous claims as to its incredible rejuvenating properties.

Raw Honey (Wildflower, Unfiltered, Uncooked Honey) - Bursting with live enzymes, antioxidants, B vitamins, potassium, antimicrobial properties, and alkalizing and healing qualities, this type of honey from fruit trees is a superfood. Despite many misconstrued notions, honey does not affect blood sugar levels directly. In its raw state, it is safe for most consumers if monitored correctly. Moreover, its antimicrobial properties play a great role in preventing growth and propagation of many microorganisms. Wildflower honey acts as an incredible pre- and pro- biotic as it aids in the formation of "good bacteria" or intestinal flora—a key element in the achievement of a healthy gastrointestinal tract. Always be cautious with any concentrated form of sugar, and be mindful of your specific case.

Bee Pollen – It's one of the most complete foods on the planet. One ounce of pollen per day has enough value to sustain life completely by itself. It has amazing anti-aging, regenerative, and revitalizing properties. It promotes higher mental efficiency, focus, power, and concentration, and can assist as an antidepressant by lifting mood. It has all essential amino acids (complete protein) that elevate athletic ability, body building, increased endurance, and recovery. It helps to activate the thymus gland (overall vitality) and strengthen overall immunity. It helps to reverse anemic conditions as it builds red blood corpuscles and hemoglobin. Bee pollen is also a great tool for weight management. It assists with sexual vigor (impotence/sperm count/performance), it can increase self-confidence, and it provides menopause relief. It protects the body from dehydration and skin disorders.

Propolis – It is a resin-like mix that bees collect from sap and flower and tree buds. It is often referred to as Russian penicillin because it has shown to be quite effective in not only protecting the hive from pests and intruders, but also assists in enhancing our immunity. It has antimicrobial, antiviral, and antiseptic properties that serve to enhance our overall shielding from pathogens we are exposed to every day. Next time your throat itches, mix some propolis with honey and take as medicine. It's included in the Antidote formula because it completes the full protective and nourishing complex with the wild honey, pollen, and royal jelly.

Shilajit – This is a highly priced Ayurvedic herb. It's a concentrated mineral pitch that is harvested from extreme altitudes in the Himalayan Mountains (approximately 3,000–13,000 feet). It's first broken down by massive microbial processes from substances derived from ancient ecosystems. It has very high concentrations of at least 84 organic minerals. It's complex nutrient and constituent profile has been speculated to help in many diverse body functions. From digestion, elimination, detox, and overall endocrine and nervous system function, shilajit is often considered a panacea for many. It should be noted that it has been utilized for thousands of years in the Ayurvedic system of care.

Chapter 7:

Crafting a Shake

The Last Five Shakes You'll Ever Need

Today, easy access to information and media has created infinite possibilities as to what we can create in our kitchen. From gourmet, simple-to-make, Mediterranean, or any cooking style desired, there is a sea of recipe books, blogs, and video tutorials online. There are also many recipes available for smoothies, juices, and shakes. A lot of these have many elements in common. Some of the approaches have value, yet most lack innovation and originality.

I have been successfully creating shakes both at home and in a high-traffic restaurant environment for over 10 years. I have tried many things and have developed my own approach, techniques, and recipes. At the end of the day, this is why this book exists. My intent is to share what I have learned. I want to pass on a meaningful system for creating shakes, elixirs, and truly nutritional drinks that stand out. Here are some insights based on my experience as to what I feel works versus what often misses the mark.

In Chapter 4, we went over how to choose the right base. Once again, starting with a strong base truly is a key component that should not be overlooked. It can make or break your final product. I have tried water, fruit juice, store-bought milk and milk alternatives, fresh coconut water, and even cold-pressed juice. Again, some of these work for fruit smoothies, frappes, slushies, etc. I am not too keen on using any of these for smoothies, however, because when I choose to drink something that has calories, it better have nutrient-dense elements in it as well. The base is important, and I do recommend re-reading the section on it if necessary.

A shake is defined in many ways. It is actually used quite a bit in the bodybuilding circles. However, putting huge amounts of inexpensive protein powders with water in a plastic blender bottle hardly constitutes a shake in my book.

Another common and very popular approach is the use and concept of green smoothies. Although I respect and appreciate the idea behind it—especially since it is a more nutritious approach to smoothies—I'm not a fan of this strategy. I never use them, no matter how good kale, spinach, and the other greens look on paper. These are all foods that I enjoy by preparing them properly with a meal. Most of the time, the recommendation is to throw those vegetables in a blender raw with lots of fruit and maybe a few powders here and there. Perhaps this might be a good way of getting some additional fiber, but some of these harder-to-digest greens need a better mechanism to extract the minerals. Cooking, dehydrating, marinating, and other processes like long-term lacto-fermentation tend to be better when it comes to digesting and assimilating the full spectrum of nutrients from these foods. Last, green smoothies, simply put, just don't taste great. In my book, they don't have the nutritional punch that is claimed, and you need way too much fruit to even make them somewhat palatable. These drinks typically miss the rich and complete flavor profile of a well-designed super shake. Again, I'm not a fan.

Probably the most ordered and popular smoothie in most retail establishments is the good old strawberry-banana combo. I have only one basic thing to say about that: *boring!* For the most part, this inexpensive option is a simple mix of fruit juice, frozen fruit, and, you guessed it, additional sugar to top it off. Whether they use white processed sugar, cheap honey, or some other type of highly processed syrup, none of these make for a nutritional drink.

Other ways that shakes are typically made involve mixes with milk, soy milk, yogurt or Greek yogurt, and the now more available grain, nut, seed, and coconut boxed milk alternatives. Again, some of these are moving in a better direction, but they still miss the mark, especially if people are still using soy milk or conventional, pasteurized, homogenized, non-organic milk. The quality and proper use of ingredients really does make a big difference.

Finally, I would like to touch upon the more purist approach to making smoothies. These shakes typically have a mixture of dates and cashews as the base. Then they have some vegan- or Paleo-type protein added, along with frozen fruit and more nuts. And some people also add a blend of a gajillion superfood powders. Almost always after consuming these concoctions, a person tends to feel pretty uncomfortable. They tend to have lots of gas and feel digestive distress. I'm trying to avoid this by using all the elements presented in this book as a complete package of sorts. These types of smoothies often come out of the more extreme dietary sects where standards are extremely high and too many restrictions and rules prevail. I began my journey in one of those camps and traveled all the way to the other extreme. After life took me on that roller coaster, I came out with a more balanced approach where I pretty much took the best of all worlds. Now my intention is to offer my own spin and go beyond with what I've learned.

So, crafting the best shake requires a simple formula that is somewhat tweaked based on the outcome desired. All shakes begin with a balanced and substantial base—the ones we mentioned before. What makes a shake a shake is that it needs to be thick and somewhat decadent. This is why so many people use frozen bananas. It makes for a decent ice cream consistency. I'm not a fan of banana. I don't care for this way-too-hybridized and nutritionally unimpressive ingredient. I do understand, however, that the ice cream consistency should be there for a good shake. So, my secret weapon? Mamey.

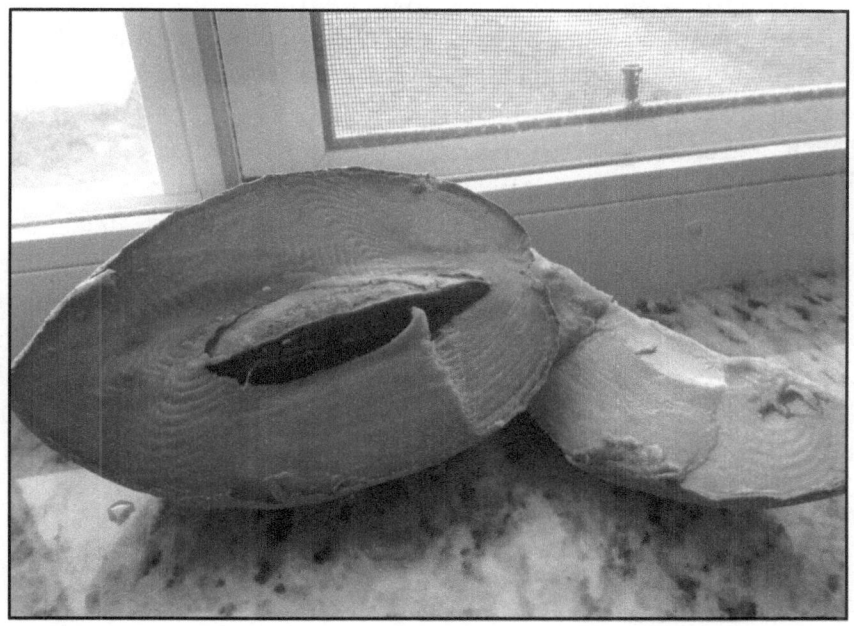

Mamey is an amazing and delicious tropical fruit from the sapote family. Imagine a mix between papaya and avocado in texture and flavor. Its bright, rich orange color makes for a vibrant stand-alone shake, but its texture is what's king. It's been my secret weapon for years. The best way to use mamey is to cut after proper ripening (when it has a very soft husk) and freeze it for shakes.

The best place to get mamey is in tropical stores in areas where it grows. These are Latin American cities and, of course, in Miami, Florida. If fresh is not available, they do sell decent frozen mamey in certain supermarkets and Latin-type stores. If this is not an option because it's not local or not available, don't sweat it. Papaya from Brazil or Latin America is more readily available and also works. A little avocado and papaya mixed together also does the job. And if all else fails, or if you don't care for frozen fruit, Irish moss gel or a nice hydrated chia seed "pudding" with the consistency of rice or tapioca pudding can thicken up a shake like the best of them.

If a simple smoothie is desired, then after the base a nice combo of frozen fruits can be blended together with a little ice and possibly some palm sugar. Some examples are acai, mamey, guanabana, or papaya with berries like strawberry, raspberry, and blueberries. See some of the recipes for further ideas.

The shake, although it begins with the same base concept, gets a little bit more creative and at times a little more strategic. So, with that comes my idea of the last five shakes you'll ever need. The reason I approached it in this way is because each one of these represents a slightly varied technique that can be used with a few different ingredients plugged in here and there. I will elaborate on each one with a recipe as the example to follow. So here we go.

1. Vanilla Supreme

This shake is one of my favorites. It's not my most favorite because it has no chocolate and sometimes I'm a chocolate freak. It's incredible, however, and my second go-to shake. With this particular shake, I attempt to recreate that decadent and rich 1950s-style vanilla ice cream milk shake that so many of us have salivated over in the past. The difference here is that this one can actually be used as a meal replacement without the guilt and with possibly the most nutritious elements you can imagine. We are using coconut or Wild Milk as the base, true six-hour bovine colostrum, grass-fed whey, some wildflower raw honey, pasture-raised egg yolks, and vanilla. The trick is in how you mix it and getting the right balance. So, more or less, for 1 (16-ounce) serving, this is how it goes:

 - 1 cup of ice
 - ¼–½ cup canned coconut milk, or about ¾ cup of Wild Milk (any flavor)
 - 3–6 tablespoons colostrum
 - 2–3 tablespoons of the whole, grass-fed whey protein
 - 1–3 teaspoons wild honey.
 - 2 egg yolks
 - 1 teaspoon vanilla extract or ½ teaspoon pure vanilla powder

Blend slowly and enjoy this incredible treat of a meal.

Note: *Make sure the honey lies right on top of all the powders and doesn't touch the ice. This way, once you blend, the honey won't stick to any of the frozen bits and will blend throughout. As is, the shake should be sweet enough, but feel free to add 5–10 drops of liquid stevia if desired. In addition, a good-quality collagen protein can be added to add some extra nutrition (approximately 1 tablespoon is usually good). This shake is mostly a strong hormone builder, and it's great to build and strengthen the body. Again, the technique can be used to make similar shake versions like a frozen berry,* *chocolate, a green version using spirulina and chlorella, or even a peanut butter-type flavor using a little nut or sunflower seed butter. But for a straight-up, jacked-up vanilla shake flavor, simply follow the recipe as is.*

2. Energy Super Blast

Everyone always wants more energy, and this shake definitely delivers. This one is actually my favorite—as I mentioned, I like chocolate. I almost always use it as my breakfast starter. So, as with all the shakes, I begin with my signature Wild Milk. I add pure cacao (chocolate) powder, grass-fed whey, colostrum, maca, cordyceps, and grade B maple syrup or palm nectar. I don't typically need or care for coffee, but this shake can be altered by cutting the Wild Milk in half and substituting the other half with a high-quality coffee. It gives a nice mocha feeling to it. So here's the usual recipe, more or less:

- 1½ cups Wild Milk
- ½ cups frozen mamey, (if no mamey is available use 2 tablespoons almond butter or chia gel, to thicken the shake)
- 2 heaping tablespoons cacao powder
- 2–4 tablespoons colostrum
- 1–2 tablespoons grass-fed whey
- 1 teaspoon maca
- 1 teaspoon cordyceps powder, or a dropper full of tincture
- 1tablespoon maple syrup or palm nectar
- ½ cup ice

Blend all ingredients together smoothly, except the whey. Once blended, add the whey and quickly pulse on low. Serve and enjoy.

This shake will get you going and make you focused, energized, and very productive. Feel free to add 1–2 teaspoons MCT oil, (Medium Chain Triglycerides from coconut), vanilla, extra almond butter, or substitute Irish moss for mamey.

3. Superior Immunity

This shake was created to boost immunity. Here, I introduce a valuable technique and concept that typically assists the liver in digesting fat. In this way, it helps build on the immune factors of the ingredients. To start the shake, I emulsify coconut oil with sunflower seed lecithin, a tiny bit of honey, and a little hot water. Making an emulsion, although not a mandatory practice, is quite helpful in making essential oils and fats more miscible with water and easier to digest. For this, we use non-GMO lecithin to bind the elements together. Lecithin is quite helpful in emulsifying the mixture with honey, as well. This is a great practice as it promotes an ideal intake of essential fatty acids and aids in the flow of bile in the body. To emulsify any drink or mixture, simply take an oil of choice (e.g., olive, ghee, or coconut) and blend with a bit of lecithin and warm water—this also works well with honey in the mixture. Again, lecithin is a great fortifying food. Lecithin from non-GMO soy or sunflower seed is rich in inositol and choline, which are elements that nourish the brain and overall cell function. It's also extremely bioavailable in pasture-raised egg yolks. So, to the shake:

- 1 tablespoon wildflower raw honey
- 1–2 tablespoons coconut oil
- 1–2 teaspoons sunflower seed lecithin powder. If working with granulated lecithin, always use a bit more (in this example, it would be about 1 tablespoon).
- ¼ cup hot water.

Blend on high for 30 seconds, or until the mix is emulsified or fully blended.

4. Hormone Blast

This super shake has some of the most androgen-type and hormone-building complexes available in the natural world. I won't go into too much detail, but let's say one night I drank this shake before turning in, and the next morning it was all smiles through and through.

- 1½ cups Wild Milk, or ¼–½ cup canned coconut milk with ¾ cup water
- 1 tablespoon almond butter or chia gel
- 1–2 tablespoons colostrum
- 1–2 tablespoons grass-fed whey protein
- 2 pasture-raised egg yolks
- 1–2 teaspoons pine pollen powder
- 1 teaspoon maca
- 1–2 teaspoons coconut oil or grass-fed ghee
- 1 tablespoon palm nectar or wild honey
- ½ cup ice

Blend all ingredients and enjoy.

5. Wild Berry Cream

This is a body builder and a shake that can be modified quite a bit into a similar nondairy option.

- 1 cup grass-fed raw milk
- ½ cup grass-fed raw yogurt
- 1–2 tablespoons grass-fed raw heavy cream
- 1–2 tablespoons colostrum
- 1 tablespoon grass-fed, whole-whey protein
- 1 tablespoon goji
- ½ cup frozen berries of choice
- 1 tablespoon organic pure cane crystals

Blend all ingredients and enjoy.

The milk can be omitted, and coconut milk combo with water or any flavor of Wild Milk can be used instead.

Chapter 8:

Recipes

Not Your Average Smoothie

Notes:

Any time lecithin is placed in a recipe, it will typically be used to emulsify, as mentioned in the previous chapter. A lot of times, you can simply just add the lecithin and blend all together, but I like to think blending it first gives the shake a slight benefit. The truth is that I'm most likely being romantic about it, but what the heck? I don't think it hurts.

Most recipes here will have, for easy readability and to avoid being repetitive, the Wild Milk as the suggested base. Always feel free to use the other two main recommendations listed in the base sections—any of the instant nut milks or ¼–½ cup canned coconut milk with 1 cup pristine water. Also use any of the nut milks offered here in the following recipes, as well.

NUT MILKS

Brazil Nut Milk

Makes approximately 7 cups

- ¾ cup Brazil nuts
- 6 cups water
- ⅛–¼ cup uncooked, unfiltered, wildflower honey, coconut palm nectar, or maple syrup
- 1½ tablespoons coconut oil
- 1 tablespoon non-GMO lecithin granules, or 1 teaspoon liquid or powdered lecithin
- ¼ cup warm water
- 1½ tablespoons Irish moss gel
- 1 teaspoon sun-dried sea salt
- 1 tablespoon vanilla extract, or 1 teaspoon vanilla powder (optional)

In a high-speed or regular blender, blend nuts and 6 cups of water thoroughly, and pour through a nut bag or strainer into a large bowl. Combine honey (or sweetener of choice), coconut oil/butter, lecithin, and ¼ cup water in the blender, and make a blended emulsion. Add salt and Irish moss gel, and blend again. Pour the mixture into the bowl with milk, whisk, and pour into a pitcher.

Notes:
This milk can be made with almonds, pumpkin seeds, macadamia nuts, or any other nut and seed as preferred.
With any of these milk recipes, you can also forgo the sweetener and simply make an unsweetened milk, or lower it significantly by using lucuma powder or a wild liquid stevia.

"New Revolutionary" Approach

Why so revolutionary? Simply stated, this next recipe represents an altered version of making nut milk. It's fast, it's easy, cleanup is a cinch, and no more nut milk bags.

Easy "Buttermilk"

Makes approximately 7 cups

- ¼ cup Brazil nut butter, coconut butter, or nut/seed butter of choice
- 6 cups water
- ¼ cup uncooked, unfiltered wildflower honey, coconut palm nectar, or maple syrup
- 1 tablespoon coconut oil/butter
- 1 tablespoon non-GMO lecithin granules, or 1 teaspoon liquid or powdered lecithin
- 1 teaspoon sun-dried sea salt
- 1 teaspoon vanilla powder, or 1 tablespoon vanilla extract
- 1½ tablespoon Irish moss gel (optional)
- 1 teaspoon tocotrienols (optional)

Blend all ingredients thoroughly, chill, and enjoy.

Coconut "Chicha" Milk

Makes approximately 7 cups

- ½–1 cup coconut flakes
- 7 cups water
- ¼ cup uncooked, unfiltered, wildflower honey, coconut palm nectar, or maple syrup
- 1 tablespoon coconut oil/butter
- 1½ tablespoon non-GMO lecithin
- 1½ tablespoon Irish moss gel
- 1 teaspoon sun-dried sea salt
- 1 teaspoon tocotrienols
- 1 teaspoon vanilla powder, or 1 tablespoon vanilla extract
- Blend the coconut flakes and water, strain, and blend remainder of ingredients thoroughly. Chill and enjoy.

Notes:

To *lower carbohydrate intake in any or all of these drinks, you can do one of two things:*

1) Start with an unsweetened nut milk of choice, instead of the sweetened ones.

2) Play with a smaller amount of sweetener and bring the sweet factor up by using a liquid stevia with a tiny pinch of living salt.

For extra protein in any of these drinks, you can also add 1 or 2 tablespoons of sprouted, cultured, live, organic brown rice protein, grass-fed whey protein (if digestible), or, if it resonates with you, 1 or 2 pasture-raised raw eggs.

If lecithin is not your thing, you don't need to use it in any of these drinks. Again, it is included here as a fortifying food to enhance digestion and brain function—especially if you do not use lecithin-rich eggs in your diet.

One last thing: a lot of these recipes have frozen mamey as a key ingredient. If it is not available or local to your area, you can always substitute with 2-3 tablespoons of Irish moss gel or 2-4 tablespoon of chia seed gel.

WUGUP (Where U Getting Ur Protein) Shake

Makes approximately 14 ounces

- 10 ounces Wild Milk of choice
- ¼ cup frozen mamey, ¼ cup Irish moss gel, or 3 tablespoons chia gel
- 1 tablespoon cacao nibs
- 1 tablespoon cacao powder
- 1 tablespoon goji berries
- 1 teaspoon bee pollen
- 1 tablespoon grass-fed whey or plant-based protein of choice (add an extra tablespoon for more protein if desired)
- 1 teaspoon spirulina
- ½–1 tablespoon raw, unfiltered, wildflower honey, palm nectar, or lucuma
- 1 tablespoon coconut butter
- 3–5 ice cubes
- 1 teaspoon Oceans Alive Phytoplankton or E3 Live Blue-Green Algae (optional)

Blend all ingredients, except ice, in a high-speed or regular blender.

Add honey right before blending so it does not stick to the blender walls. Blend, add ice, and blend again. Enjoy.

MPTWN Shake (More Protein for Those Who Need It)

- 1½ cup Wild Milk of choice
- 2–3 tablespoons coconut cream
- 2–4 tablespoons grass-fed whey or plant-based protein of choice
- 1–2 tablespoons frozen mamey, papaya, chia gel, or Irish moss gel
- 1–2 teaspoons lucuma powder
- 5–8 drops liquid stevia, or 1–2 teaspoons wild honey
- ½ teaspoon vanilla powder, or 1 teaspoon extract
- Pinch of sun-dried sea salt
- 4–6 drops orange or lemon flavor (optional)

Blend all ingredients, except ice, in a high-speed or regular blender. Add ice, blend again, and enjoy.

John's Cacao Shake

Makes approximately 17 ounces

- 12 ounces nut milk of choice
- ¼ cup frozen mamey or Irish moss gel
- 1–2 tablespoons raw cacao powder
- 1 tablespoon raw cacao nibs
- ½–1 tablespoon raw, unfiltered, wildflower honey or raw (clear) agave
- 3–5 ice cubes (optional)

Blend all ingredients, except ice, in a high-speed or regular blender. Add ice, blend again, and enjoy.

Notes:
Add honey right before blending so it does not stick to the blender walls. Blend, add ice, and blend again. Enjoy.

If you are a dark chocolate lover, add an extra tablespoon of raw cacao powder. Insane!

GojiOxidant

Makes 16 ounces

- 1½ cup Wild Milk of choice
- 2 tablespoons goji
- ½ cup mamey
- 1 tablespoon lucuma
- 1 tablespoons grass-fed whey or plant-based protein of choice
- 1½ tablespoons palm sugar
- 4 ice cubes

Blend all ingredients, except ice, in a high-speed or regular blender. Add ice, blend again, and enjoy.

Supreme Green

Makes 16 ounces

- 1½ cups Wild Milk
- ½ cup mamey
- 1 teaspoon spirulina
- 1 teaspoon chlorella
- 1 tablespoon lucuma
- 1 tablespoon grass-fed whey or plant-based protein of choice
- 1 tablespoon palm sugar
- 4 ice cubes

Blend all ingredients, except ice, in a high-speed or regular blender except ice. Add ice, blend again, and enjoy.

Mocha

Makes 16 ounces

- 1 cup Wild Milk
- ½ cup mamey
- 1 teaspoons reishi coffee
- 1 teaspoon mesquite
- 1 teaspoon cacao
- 1½ tablespoons palm sugar
- 3 cubes ice

Blend all ingredients, except ice, in a high-speed or regular blender except ice. Add ice, blend again, and enjoy.

Basic Fruit Smoothie with Variations

Makes approximately 16 ounces
Base:

- – ½–1 tablespoon uncooked, unfiltered, wildflower honey, palm nectar, or lucuma
- – 1–2 tablespoons coconut oil
- – 1 tablespoon non-GMO lecithin granules
- – ¼ cup pristine water
- – 10 ounces (or 1 ¼ cups) milk of choice
- – 1 cup frozen fruit of choice

Examples:

1. ½ cup mango + ½ cup papaya
2. ½ cup acai + ½ cup papaya or passion fruit
3. 1 cup mixed berries
4. ¾ cup mamey + ¼ cup papaya
5. ½ cup passion fruit + ½ cup papaya or mango

- – Add: tocotrienols or maca for added nutrition (optional)

Make emulsion in the blender with first four ingredients. Add the remaining ingredients and blend. Add ice, blend again, and enjoy.

> **Note:**
> *All these fruit smoothie recipes tend to be medium to high in carbohydrates, so it's wise to be cautious with these. If you're trying to lose weight, are dealing with candida, hyperglycemia, hypoglycemia, diabetes, or a metabolic type is not aligned with these foods, be mindful of tweaking or forgoing these recipes all together.*

Mamey

Makes 16 ounces

- 1½ cups Wild Milk
- 1 cup frozen mamey
- 1½ tablespoons palm sugar
- 3 ice cubes

Blend all ingredients, except ice, in a high-speed or regular blender. Add ice, blend again, and enjoy.

Acai

Makes 16 ounces

- 1½ cups Wild Milk
- 1 serving of frozen acai pulp
- ¼ - ½ cup mamey
- 1½ - 2 tablespoons palm sugar
- 3 ice cubes

Blend all ingredients, except ice, in a high-speed or regular blender. Add ice, blend again, and enjoy.

Mango

Makes 16 ounces

- 1½ cups Wild Milk
- ¾ cups frozen mango
- 1 tablespoons palm sugar
- 3 ice cubes

Blend all ingredients, except ice, in a high-speed or regular blender. Add ice, blend again, and enjoy.

Mixed Berry

Makes 16 ounces

- 1½ cups Wild Milk
- 1/2 cup frozen mamey
- ¼- 1/2 cup frozen berries
- 1-2 tablespoon palm sugar

Blend all ingredients in a high-speed or regular blender and enjoy.

Peaches and Cream Shake

Makes approximately 16 ounces

- ½–1 tablespoon uncooked, unfiltered, wildflower honey, palm nectar, or lucuma
- 1 tablespoon coconut oil
- 1 tablespoon non-GMO lecithin granules
- ¼ cup pristine water
- 1 cup nut milk of choice
- 1–2 tablespoons Irish moss gel
- 2 fresh peaches (pits removed), or 2 cups frozen peaches
- 2 dried figs, or 4 dried apricots, soaked (optional)
- Pinch cinnamon (optional)
- Drop vanilla (optional)
- Add: tocotrienols or maca for added nutrition (optional)

Make emulsion in the blender with first four ingredients. Add the remaining ingredients and blend. Add ice, blend again, and enjoy.

Creamsicle Delight

Makes 16 ounces

- ½–1 tablespoon uncooked, unfiltered, wildflower honey, palm nectar, or lucuma
- 1 tablespoon coconut oil
- 1 tablespoon non-GMO lecithin granules
- ¼ cup pristine water
- 1 cup nut milk of choice
- ½ cup frozen peaches
- 2 tablespoons cubed fresh or frozen papaya
- 1 teaspoon orange extract

Make emulsion in the blender with first four ingredients. Add the remaining ingredients and blend. Add ice, blend again, and enjoy.

Electrolyte Lemonade

Makes approximately ½ gallon

- 3 whole lemons (white pith and seeds included, but not the yellow peel)
- 1 apple or pear, cored
- 5 tablespoons unfiltered, uncooked, wildflower honey or palm nectar
- 2 tablespoons coconut oil
- 1 teaspoon sun-dried sea salt
- 5 cups pristine water
- ½-inch piece fresh ginger, or to taste (start small)

Blend all ingredients in a high-speed or regular blender.
For each serving, mix 8 ounces lemonade with 8 ounces nut milk of choice.

"NO-SUGAR" RECIPES

"No-Sugar" Nut Milk

Makes ¾ of a Gallon

- ½ cup Brazil nut butter or nut/seed butter of choice
- 10 cups water
- 2 tablespoons coconut oil
- 1½ teaspoons sea salt
- 1 tablespoon mesquite
- 1 teaspoon lecithin
- 4 tablespoons Irish moss gel (optional)
- 1 teaspoon vanilla powder
- 1 tablespoon tocotrienols
- ⅛–¼ teaspoon stevia herb, or 10 drops liquid stevia
- 1 tablespoon lakanto (optional)

Blend all ingredients in a high-speed or regular blender. If using a small blender, blend all ingredients with 4–5 cups water, and transfer to a bottle or pitcher. Add remaining water into the bottle or pitcher, and shake or stir to combine.

Mighty Macacao

Makes approximately 12 ounces

- 10 ounces "no-sugar" nut milk
- 2 tablespoons Irish moss gel
- 2 teaspoons mesquite
- 2 tablespoon maca
- 1 tablespoon coconut oil
- 1 teaspoon vanilla powder
- 1 tablespoon cacao powder
- 1 tablespoon coconut cream or extra nut butter
- 1 tablespoon tocotrienols
- 1 tablespoon lucuma
- 5 drops liquid stevia
- 3-5 cubes ice
- 2 teaspoons lakanto or xylitol (optional)

Blend all ingredients, except ice, in a high-speed or regular blender. Add ice, blend again, and enjoy.

Carobccino Drink

Makes approximately 12 ounces

- 10 ounces "no-sugar" nut milk of choice
- 2 tablespoons Irish moss or nut butter
- 1 tablespoon coconut oil
- 1 tablespoon tocotrienols
- 2 tablespoons carob powder
- 2 teaspoons mesquite
- 1 tablespoon lucuma
- ½ teaspoon vanilla powder or 1tsp extract
- 3-5 cubes ice
- Pinch of stevia herb, or 5 drops liquid stevia (optional)

Blend all ingredients, except ice, in a high-speed or regular blender. Add ice, blend again, and enjoy.

The "Green Beast" Shake

Makes approximately 16 ounces

- 1 cup "no-sugar" nut milk of choice
- 1 tablespoon E3 Live liquid, or 1–2 teaspoons powder
- 5 drops phytoplankton
- 1 handful fresh mint leaves
- 5 drops liquid stevia
- 1 teaspoon spirulina
- 1 teaspoon chlorella
- 1 handful sunflower sprouts
- 1 teaspoon coconut oil
- 1 tablespoon tocotrienols
- 1 tablespoon lucuma
- 2 teaspoons mesquite
- 3-5 cubes ice
- 1 tablespoon lakanto (optional)

Blend all ingredients, except ice, in a high-speed or regular blender. Add ice, blend again, and enjoy.

Medicinal Magic Shake

Makes approximately 16 ounces

- 1 cup "no-sugar" nut milk of choice
- 2 tablespoons coconut cream
- 1 tablespoon maca
- 1 dropper of reishi tincture
- 1 teaspoon lion's mane powder
- 1 teaspoon cordyceps powder
- 1 teaspoon vanilla powder
- 2 teaspoon carob
- 1 teaspoon mesquite
- 1 tablespoon tocotrienols
- 5 drops liquid stevia
- 3-5 cubes ice
- 2 teaspoons lakanto (optional)

Blend all ingredients, except ice, in a high-speed or regular blender. Add ice, blend again, and enjoy.

Note:
  For *medicinal mushroom activation, you can also do a chaga/reishi decoction concentrate and use this in your recipe. You can also use a mixed blend formula such as Surthriva's or Paul Stamet's Mycommunity product caps (opening the capsules and adding the powder inside). Dragon Herbs and Jing herbs are also good.*

HEALING WITH HERBS: ELIXIRS & SUPER DRINKS

This small section is inspired by a wonderful wave of increased awareness regarding the power of herbs. There is a growing community of supercharged individuals who are grasping strategies to use medicinal herbs and wild food—especially alkaloid constituents—to extract powerful value in the hidden gems that nature offers us every day.

I want to extend credit and gratitude to all the cutting-edge individuals who have paved the way and put forth an incredible energy shift toward the value of alchemy and a natural "flying high" mentality. When it comes to nutrition, the value of water and getting the most from what we have available is truly a beautiful thing.

What follows is an example, along with some ideas on how to incorporate elixir and herbal concoctions into one's lifestyle without having to necessarily follow a recipe. I am of the mindset that these specific types of drinks are meant to be created with a very unique artistic approach, innovation, and an element of magical inspiration. Therefore, I will share my basic technique with ideas on how to extract these herbal elements. Also, I will mention the herbs and compounds I like to work with the most.

Decoctions and Infusions: Base Ideas

A decoction is a "slow cooking" of tough herbs that usually come from tree bark, hard medicinal mushrooms, and tough dried berries (e.g., Hawthorne, schizandra, juniper). These elements can be prepared on a wood burning stove or a gas burner by bringing natural or pure water to a low boil for a few minutes with the herbs, and then allowing them to simmer for at least 20 minutes. Some herbs require longer extraction in order to acquire more medicine. I recommend getting to know your herbs of choice well. A slow cooker can also do the job by cooking the herbs and pristine water on low for 8–24 hours.

An infusion, or herbal tea, is one that can be made using very light heat, sun extraction, or moon extraction overnight. Infusions are usually possible with gentler flower-, petal-, or leaf-type herbs (e.g., nettle leaf, chamomile, red raspberry, and lavender).

Also, when one powders and finely sieves some of these herbs, it is very possible to also obtain a quicker and more "instant extraction" from hot water.

So, here are some ideas on my favorite elixir-type drinks:

First, the decoction/infusion bases:

1. Immune System Amazonia - cat's claw, pau d'arco, chanca piedra (break stone), nettle root and leaf, burdock and catuaba
2. Liver - milk thistle, dandelion, burdock, yellow dock, bupleurum, rhodiola, schizandra, nettle leaf
3. Ayurvedic Bunch - tribulus, shilijit, holy basil, bacopa, mucuna, amla berry, ashwaganda, turmeric
4. Immunity Mushroom - reishi, cordyceps, lion's mane, shiitake, maitake, chaga
5. Daoist Approach - reishi, he shou wu, schizandra, goji, astragalus

In deciding the amount of herbs to use for extractions and teas, I always like to use intuition. A good measure, however, is about 1–2 teaspoons of herbs per 8 ounces of water. Some herbs and compounds are stronger than others. Also, when it comes to some of the more medicinal adaptogenic herbs, I'm one who tends to put more compounds/amounts into my own personal concoctions. This, of course, is a personal choice, and my advice is always to follow your experience, intuition, and your body's own perfect intelligence above all else.

So here's a great example of an awesome drink I like to take every so often. Remember, it is always good to rotate things when working with herbs. Do things more on a rest/active cycle instead of bringing the same stuff in every day. So, here we go:

1. Make your super tea base (in this case, Immune System Amazonia)
2. Strain about 8 ounces of the super tea into a blender and add the following more or less in these ratios:

- An extra cup or so nut milk of choice
- 2–3 tablespoons coconut cream
- 1–2 tablespoons colostrum
- 1 tablespoon Irish moss gel or Brazil nut butter
- 1 tablespoon goji berries
- 1 tablespoon cacao powder
- 1 tablespoon cacao nibs
- 1 tablespoon tocotrienols
- ¼ teaspoon nutmeg
- ¼–½ teaspoon cinnamon
- ¼ teaspoon sun-dried sea salt
- 1 teaspoon vanilla powder
- ½–1 teaspoon turmeric
- 1 teaspoon lucuma
- 1 teaspoon mesquite
- 1–2 teaspoons wild honey or yacon syrup (optional)
- 1–2 tablespoons grass-fed whey or plant protein (optional)

Enjoy and fly.

Remember, the drink listed here is one of the many types that we have in our wonderful day and age. Also, remember to always study the herbs, especially if the subject of pregnancy applies to you.

Notes:

The bases used here also make extremely great and powerful super-soup bases. Some recipes will follow in the soup section as well.

Another idea for getting quick and easy alchemical ingredients into a drink is to incorporate either homemade tinctures, or find a reputable brand of liquid tinctured herbs.

And yes, I said no recipes needed, but what the heck? Here's a quick list of recipe ideas to play with for tonic drinks:

ImmunoShield

- 12 ounces base (gynostemma)
- 1½ tablespoons grass-fed whey
- 1 tablespoon colostrum
- 1 tablespoon lucuma
- 1/2 teaspoon reishi tincture
- 1 teaspoon cordyceps powder
- 1 teaspoon chaga tincture
- 1 teaspoon astragalus
- 1 tablespoon coconut concentrate

Blend and enjoy.

Genius Rising

- 12 ounces base (gynostemma)
- 1 tablespoon grass-fed whey
- 1 tablespoon lucuma
- 1 tablespoon cacao
- ¼ teaspoon blue-green algae
- ¼ teaspoon mucuna
- 1/4 teaspoon bacopa
- 1 tablespoon MCT (medium chain triglycerides from coconut) oil

Blend and enjoy.

All Mighty

- 12 ounces base (gynostemma)
- 2 tablespoons grass-fed whey
- 1 teaspoon maca
- 1 teaspoon cordyceps powder
- 1 teaspoon pine pollen
- 1 dropper Jing herbs Shen Nong's Ginseng
- ¼ teaspoon tribulus
- 1 tablespoon coconut concentrate
- 1 teaspoon polyrachis powder

Blend and enjoy.

Nerve Endings

- 12 ounces base (gynostemma)
- 1 tablespoon grass-fed whey
- ½ teaspoon holy basil
- 1 tablespoon colostrum
- 1 tablespoon tocotrienols
- 1 tablespoon chia gel
- 1–2 teaspoon MCT (medium chain triglycerides from coconut) oil

Blend and enjoy.

Rebuild-a-Tissue

- 12 ounces base (gynostemma)
- 1-2 tablespoons grass-fed whey
- 1 tablespoon cacao
- 1 teaspoon mesquite
- 1 teaspoon polyrachis powder
- 1 teaspoon cordyceps powder
- 1-2 tablespoons collagen powder
- ¼ teaspoon blue-green algae
- 1 tablespoon coconut concentrate

Blend and enjoy.

Love My Liver

- 12 ounces Liver tea (burdock, dandelion, yellow dock, milk thistle)
- 1 – 2 tablespoons grass-fed whey
- 1 teaspoon chai spice
- 1 tablespoon coconut concentrate

Blend and enjoy.

The following are examples of some other sun-and-summer type teas:

Tummy Ease

Makes approximately ½ gallon

- — 2 tablespoons dried peppermint
- — 2 tablespoons dried fennel
- — 1 tablespoon fresh ginger
- — 1 teaspoon clove
- — ½–1 cup wild honey, or 10 drops wild Amazon stevia

Steep tea in approximately 14 ounces of hot water in a hermetically sealed mason jar for a few hours in the sun, or on the counter overnight. Strain and pour into a ½-gallon jug.

Add softened wild honey or stevia, and fill remainder of the vessel with pristine water.

Refrigerate or enjoy over ice.

This tea is an excellent choice to relieve stomach discomfort, alleviate gas and bloating, and ease digestion.

Easy Going

Makes approximately ½ gallon

- — 2 tablespoons red raspberry loose leaf
- — 2 tablespoons chamomile loose leaf
- — 1 tablespoon lavender loose leaf
- — ½–1 cup wild honey, or 10 drops liquid stevia

Steep tea in approximately 14 ounces of hot water in a hermetically sealed mason jar for a few hours in the sun, or on the counter overnight. Strain and pour into a ½-gallon jug.

Add softened wild honey or stevia, and fill remainder of the vessel with natural spring or pure water.

Refrigerate or enjoy over ice.

This particular mix is meant to act as a relaxer and nervous system calmative.

Ruby Red Tea

Makes approximately ½ gallon

- — 3 tablespoons dried honeybush leaves
- — 2 tablespoons dried or whole red hibiscus leaves
- — ½–1 cup wild honey, or 10 drops liquid stevia

Steep tea in approximately 14 ounces of hot water in a hermetically sealed mason jar for a few hours in the sun, or on the counter overnight. Strain and pour into a ½-gallon jug.

Add softened wild honey or stevia, and fill remainder of the vessel with natural spring or pure water.

Refrigerate or enjoy over ice.

This amazing fruit-punch-like tea is extremely powerful for keeping a healthy circulatory system.

Ginger Lemonade

Makes approximately ½ gallon

- 3 lemons, juiced
- 1–2 (1-inch) pieces fresh ginger
- 1 teaspoon sun-dried sea salt
- ½ cup wild honey

Steep finely chopped or grated fresh ginger in approximately 14 ounces of hot water in a hermetically sealed mason jar for a few hours in the sun, or on the counter overnight. Strain and pour into a ½-gallon jug. For an instant tea, you can also blend the ginger straight in the blender with the water and strain.

Add lemon juice, salt, and wild honey or stevia, and fill remainder of the vessel with natural spring or pure water.

Refrigerate or enjoy over ice.

Green Tea

Makes approximately ½ gallon

- 3 tablespoon dried green tea leaves
- ⅛–¼ cup wild honey, or 10 drops liquid stevia

Steep tea in approximately 14 ounces of hot water in a hermetically sealed mason jar for a few hours in the sun, or on the counter overnight. Strain and pour into a ½-gallon jug.

Add softened wild honey or stevia, and fill remainder of the vessel with natural spring or pure water.

Refrigerate or enjoy over ice.

Green tea is known the world over to have powerful tannins and antioxidant elements that support a healthier body.

SOUPS AND STEWS

"Sancocho" Soup

Makes 1 serving

- 3 tablespoons tomato powder
- 2 tablespoons fresh pumpkin seeds, ground
- 1 teaspoon turmeric
- 2 handfuls fresh cilantro
- 1 handful fresh parsley
- 2 tablespoons chopped cucumber
- 4 tablespoons chopped celery
- 1 teaspoon sun-dried sea salt
- 1 teaspoon paprika
- ½ teaspoon cumin
- 1 tablespoon olive oil
- 2 teaspoons apple cider vinegar
- 1 tablespoon lemon juice
- ½ avocado, cubed
- 2 tablespoons red onion
- 2 tablespoons chopped burdock
- 2 tablespoons chopped sunchoke
- 1–1½ cups warm water or broth
- 4 tablespoons cooked shiitake or oyster mushrooms (optional)

Blend all ingredients and enjoy warm.

Sea Veggie Medley Soup

Makes 1 serving

- ¾ cup soaked wakame, chopped
- 2–4 tablespoons red onion
- 4 tablespoons chopped cucumber
- 4 tablespoons chopped celery
- 1 handful sprouts
- 1 handful fresh cilantro
- 1 handful fresh parsley
- 1 teaspoon kelp
- 1 teaspoon salt
- 1 tablespoon fresh black sesame seed
- 1 handful dulse
- 1 cup warm water or broth
- 1 tablespoon olive oil
- 2 teaspoons apple cider vinegar
- 1 handful arugula
- 1 handful romaine
- 1 nori sheet, shredded
- ½ lemon (after blending)
- 5 drops phytoplankton
- ½ teaspoon jalapeno flakes (optional)

Blend all ingredients and enjoy warm.

Most Mighty Stew

Makes 1 serving

- 1 teaspoon dulse
- 5 tablespoons chopped celery
- 1 handful sprouts
- 1 handful fresh cilantro
- 1 handful fresh parsley
- 2 tablespoons tomato powder
- 2 – 4 tablespoons sunflower seeds
- Pinch black pepper
- 1 teaspoon sea salt
- ½ teaspoon turmeric
- 2 tablespoons avocado
- ½ teaspoon mesquite
- 10 ounces warm water or broth
- 1 handful wakame
- 2 tablespoons chopped zucchini
- 2 tablespoons chopped red onion
- 1 - 4 tablespoons chia seeds
- 1 tablespoon olive oil
- 2 teaspoons apple cider vinegar
- 1 tablespoon maca
- 1 handful arugula
- 1 teaspoon oregano
- 1 handful fresh basil
- 1 tablespoon nutritional yeast flakes (optional)

Blend all ingredients if desiring a creamy stew.

Asparagus Cream Soup

Makes 2 servings

- 1 cup warm nut milk of choice
- 2 tablespoons nutritional yeast flakes
- 2 tablespoons Irish moss gel, or ½ avocado
- 1 teaspoon salt
- 1 teaspoon apple cider vinegar
- 1 tablespoon olive oil
- ½ cup warm water
- 1 cup chopped, lightly steamed asparagus
- ½ cup zucchini
- ¼–½ avocado
- 1 pinch black pepper
- 1 teaspoon tocotrienols
- 1 teaspoon maca (optional)

Blend all ingredients and enjoy.

> **Note:**
>
> *If you wish to avoid possible goitrogens and have a smoother and warm soup, lightly steaming the asparagus is more than acceptable. This applies also to all the members of the brassica and mustard families, and other wild green edibles that may present challenges with the breakdown of the cellulose (plant cell wall).*

Curry Cream Soup

Makes 1 serving

- ½ cup soft, steamed butternut squash or sweet potato
- 2 tablespoons chopped celery
- 3 tablespoons chopped zucchini
- 2 tablespoons nutritional yeast flakes
- 2 tablespoons chopped bell pepper
- 1 tablespoon chopped red onion
- 1 teaspoon sea salt
- 1 teaspoon apple cider vinegar
- 1 teaspoon curry powder
- ½ teaspoon turmeric
- 2 teaspoon coconut oil
- 8–10 ounces warm water or broth
- ½ avocado (optional, for extra thickness)

Bland all ingredients and enjoy.

Sun-Dried Tomato Soup Broth

Makes approximately 32 ounces

- 1 cup water or nut milk of choice
- ½ cup Irish moss gel
- 2 tablespoons Italian seasoning
- 2 tablespoons oregano
- 1 clove garlic
- 1 teaspoon sun-dried sea salt
- ½ cup pristine water or broth
- 1½ cup sun-dried tomatoes
- 1 tablespoon lemon juice
- ⅛ cup olive oil
- ¼ cup nutritional yeast flakes (optional)

Soak sun-dried tomatoes for about 15 minutes. Blend all ingredients, except sun-dried tomatoes. Add sun-dried tomatoes and blend again.

Note:
Feel free to substitute the sun-dried tomatoes (for this or any tomato recipe) with 2–4 tablespoons of lycopene-rich and delicious super-tomato powder.

Chunky Tomato Veggie Soup

Makes approximately 16 ounces

- 8 ounces Sun-Dried Tomato Soup Broth
- ½ tomato, chopped
- 1 tablespoon pine nuts
- 1 tablespoon chopped celery
- 1 tablespoon chopped bell pepper
- 1 tablespoon chopped red onion
- 1 tablespoon olive oil (for garnish)
- 1 tablespoon chopped fresh basil
- 1 cup pristine water
- Pinch of sun-dried sea salt
- 1 teaspoon kelp powder (optional)
- Pinch cayenne pepper (optional)

Add all ingredients in a cup or bowl and mix. Alternatively, place all ingredients in a blender and blend.

Ginger-Spiced Broth

Makes approximately 40 ounces

- 2 red onions
- ¾ cup fresh ginger
- 3 cups pristine water (or a mixture of half broth and half water)
- 2 cloves garlic
- 1 tablespoon apple cider vinegar
- 1 tablespoon turmeric
- 1 tablespoon curry powder
- 1 tablespoon chili powder
- 1 tablespoon mesquite powder
- ¼ cup olive oil
- 1 teaspoon sun-dried sea salt
- 1 tablespoon lemon juice

Blend the first three ingredients really well and strain. Add the remaining ingredients and blend again.

Note:
This mix is thick and very potent. It is meant to be used primarily as a base for other soups.

Ginger Kick Soup

Makes approximately 16 ounces

- 8 ounces Ginger-Spiced Broth
- 2 tablespoons chopped tomato
- 1 tablespoon pine nuts or Brazil nuts
- 1 tablespoon chopped celery
- 1 tablespoon chopped bell pepper
- 1 tablespoon chopped red onion
- 1 tablespoon olive oil (for garnish)
- 1 tablespoon chopped fresh parsley
- Add warm water to top 16 oz container
- Pinch of sun-dried sea salt
- Pinch kelp powder (optional)
- Pinch cayenne pepper (optional)

Add all ingredients in a cup or bowl and mix. Alternatively, place all ingredients in a blender and blend.

Bell Pepper Caraway Soup

Makes approximately 25 ounces

- 2 red bell cubed peppers
- 1 tomato, chopped
- ¼ cup chopped red onion
- ¼ cup olive oil
- 1 tablespoon caraway seeds
- 2 tablespoons lemon juice
- 1 tablespoon apple cider vinegar
- 1 tablespoon wild honey
- 2 cups warm water (or a mixture of half broth and half water)
- 1 tablespoon sun-dried sea salt
- 1 teaspoon turmeric
- ¼ cup soaked walnuts
- 1 teaspoon oregano

Add all ingredients in a cup or bowl and mix. Alternatively, place all ingredients in a blender and blend.

Coconut Kefir

Slightly warm 1 quart of fresh coconut water—preferably a young green coconut—and pour into a glass container. Pour in a kefir starter that can be found at www.bodyecologydiet.com.

Next, tightly seal the vessel and allow it to sit in a dark place at room temperature (approximately 70–85 degrees F) for about 32 hours. You will notice that the coconut water becomes very cloudy and bubbles like champagne. Your kefir is ready to be consumed and stored in the fridge.

Enjoy approximately 4 ounces of the drink every day. I love this on an empty stomach after first morning's rehydration "session" with natural spring water.

Note:
If you would like to expedite this process, go to Whole Foods Market and get a shot of Inner Eco To Go coconut water kefir. Pour the whole 1-ounce bottle in a quart mason jar and top with fresh coconut water. Let sit on the counter for 24 hours and the cultured kefir is finished. Also, an already cultured batch can be recycled in this same way about six times. Simply use 2 ounces of the already cultured kefir and fill about a ½ gallon mason jar with fresh coconut water and allow to culture for 24 hours.

Simple Kefir Cocktail

- 4–6 ounces coconut water kefir
- ½ lemon, juiced and strained
- 5–10 drops liquid stevia

Pour all ingredients into a cup filled with ice. Enjoy.

Other ideas: lightly blend with a little ginger, coconut oil, lemon/lime, and a bit of lakanto or 5 drops liquid stevia.

Resources

Superfoods and Staples

WILD MILK:	www.enjoywildmilk.com
GRASS-FED WHEY:	www.wheynaturalusa.com
MARINE PHYTOPLANKTON:	http://bit.ly/1PZr8q9
PANASEEDA SEED OIL:	http://bit.ly/1Hxq2CD
SURTHRIVAL COLOSTRUM, PINE POLLEN, MEDICINAL MUSHROOMS, GRASS-FED GHEE, SCHIZANDRA:	http://bit.ly/1Pz9LBD
HONEY PRODUCTS:	Local or Health Food Stores (Look For "Raw," Wild, And Unfiltered)
BLUE-GREEN ALGAE:	e3live.com
OTHER MEDICINAL MUSHROOM PRODUCTS:	jingherbs.com, dragonherbs.com
CACAO, MACA, LUCUMA, MESQUITE:	www.andeantreasures.com
ANTIDOTE:	http://bit.ly/1IROQnG

SPIRULINA, CHLORELLA, GOJI, AND OTHER SUPERFOODS:	www.ultimatesuperfoods.com
TOCOTRIENOLS:	www.sunstarorganics.com
NUT BUTTERS:	bluemountainorganics.com
IRISH MOSS:	www.therawfoodworld.com
PRISTINE HYDRO LIVING WATER SYSTEM, ANTIDOTE, AND MAGNESIUM:	http://bit.ly/1IROQnG
FOR LOCAL, FARM-FRESH FOOD AND RAW DAIRY:	www.westonaprice.org (look for your local chapter) www.myhealthyfoodclub.com (South Florida) www.bmorganics.com
KEFIR STARTER AND LAKANTO:	www.bodyecology.com
HERBS:	www.mountainroseherbs.com www.dragonherbs.com www.jingherbs.com
BEST NUT MILK BAGS:	www.ecobags.com
FOR MASON JARS:	Visit local hardware stores, supermarkets, or places like Ross, Marshalls, and T.J. Maxx.

For a great show-and-tell version of this book and tutorial-style course, please sign up for our newsletter to get up to date information for when this program is finished. Please visit: www.howtomakesupershakes.com and sign up.

Supercharge Your Life

Thanks for reading my book! My goal is to provide you with effective tools that can easily improve your health. The strategies and techniques shared in this book offer cutting edge solutions to add value to our modern, busy lifestyles. At Schott's Wellness, we are committed to improving and continuously adding value to others. Visit our website at SchottsWellness.com and join our quest to bring forth practical rejuvenation strategies that will create evolutionary shifts, and a more balanced planet. Sign up for our newsletter today and receive our *No Need to Explain Diet Bulletin*. Also, check out HowToMakeSuperShakes.com for a video version of this book.

Thank You!

Thank you for reading this book. I do hope you found the information here to be helpful in crafting great and nutritious super shakes. I would really appreciate your feedback, so please take a moment to give a short review on Amazon. Your review will help me reach more readers, as well as help me in my future work and writing. Thank you again for reading and for taking the time to give your review!

About the Author

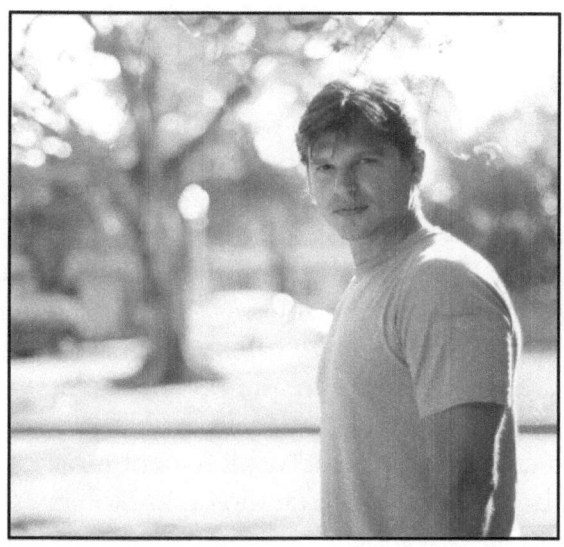

My whole life—as a boy growing up in my hometown, and now as an adult—I have always intuitively known that my mission has been to spread love and assist humanity in overcoming limits and breaking new ground. Seeing the inequities of the class system alive and well in third-world Colombia, a passion to help humanity bubbled up inside me from a very young age. As an entrepreneur in the health field, I have learned the value of hard work and excellence in everything I put forth. I pride myself on my high level of ethics and integrity in this oversaturated and confusing field of health and nutrition.

Throughout my evolution in the health field, I have run the gamut of all diets and nutritional disciplines—both time-tested and newly developed. This has brought me to a unique and more holistic place from where to educate the public on all matters of nutrition. As a gifted whole-food chef, my skill exemplifies the standard of optimal health, as well as gourmet cuisine. I am continually engaged in self-study and I am constantly absorbing new information. After 10 years of serving in the health field, and five years of being a health-food restaurant owner and general manager in Miami, Florida, I understand that this is still a very young and somewhat uncharted field. My wisdom increases with each passing day, and I appreciate all there is to learn, as I realize there is always some new facet to immerse myself in, and there are always ways to improve.

I have exposed myself to the wide spectrum of diets and food disciplines out there. I have gone through all the extremes—the SAD (Standard American Diet), veganism, vegetarianism, raw veganism, the low-carb Paleo diet, the low-fat diet, RBTI, the blood-type diet, the primal diet, and the Paleo diet. I do not have the next diet fad du jour with my name splattered all over complementary supplements to offer you. Why? Because after all these years, arduous research, and experimentations, I have found balance in eating real food in a sensible and very conscious, omnivorous manner. I believe we all benefit most from listening to our own bodies and understanding that biology is the greatest gauge. I also take advantage of some sound modern diagnostic technologies to monitor bio markers, and all biological levels, so as to minimize the guessing games. I am always on the cutting edge of whole-body and nutritional programs. Be on the cutting edge along with me and visit www.SchottsWellness.com. Own your health!